SpringerBriefs in Psychology

SpringerBriefs in Behavioral Criminology

Series Editor

Vincent B. Van Hasselt, Fort Lauderdale, FL, USA

Behavioral Criminology is a multidisciplinary approach that draws on behavioral research for the application of behavioral theories and methods to assessment, prevention, and intervention efforts directed toward violent crime and criminal behavior. Disciplines relevant to this field are criminology; criminal justice (law enforcement and corrections); forensic, correctional, and clinical psychology and psychiatry: neuropsychology, neurobiology, conflict and dispute resolution; sociology, and epidemiology. Areas of study and application include, but are not limited to: specific crimes and perpetrators (e.g., homicide and sex crimes, crimes against children, child exploitation, domestic, school, and workplace violence), topics of current national and international interest and concern (e.g., terrorism and counter terrorism, cyber crime), and strategies geared toward evaluation, identification, and interdiction with regard to criminal acts (e.g., hostage negotiation, criminal investigative analysis, threat and risk assessment). The aim of the proposed Briefs is to provide practitioners and researchers with information, data, and current best practices on important and timely topics in Behavioral Criminology. Each Brief will include a review of relevant research in the area, original data, implications of findings, case illustrations (where relevant), and recommendations for directions that future efforts might take.

More information about this series at http://www.springer.com/series/10850

Tom D. Kennedy • Elise Anello
Stephanie Sardinas • Scarlet Paria Woods

Working with Psychopathy

Lifting the Mask

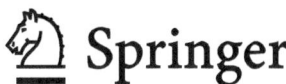 Springer

Tom D. Kennedy
College of Psychology
Nova Southeastern University
Fort Lauderdale, FL, USA

Elise Anello
College of Psychology
Nova Southeastern University
Fort Lauderdale, FL, USA

Stephanie Sardinas
College of Psychology
Nova Southeastern University
Fort Lauderdale, FL, USA

Scarlet Paria Woods
College of Psychology
Nova Southeastern University
Fort Lauderdale, FL, USA

ISSN 2192-8363   ISSN 2192-8371   (electronic)
SpringerBriefs in Psychology
ISSN 2194-1866   ISSN 2194-1874   (electronic)
SpringerBriefs in Behavioral Criminology
ISBN 978-3-030-84024-2   ISBN 978-3-030-84025-9   (eBook)
https://doi.org/10.1007/978-3-030-84025-9

This Springer imprint is published by the registered company Springer Nature Switzerland AG
The registered company address is: Gewerbestrasse 11, 6330 Cham, Switzerland

Preface

Popular cultural media such as movies, television, and books commonly characterize psychopaths as murderous monsters. They are often portrayed as intriguing and easy to recognize. In reality, an individual with psychopathic traits is much more complex and nuanced. Psychopaths can be criminals, but they may also be students, patients, clients, coworkers, or even CEOs. Murderous or not, they frequently prey on the people around them.

Psychopathy is a serious personality disorder and is represented by a specific cluster of characteristics. Although it is not an official diagnosis, it is included as a "specifier" of antisocial personality disorder in the American Psychiatric Association's (2013) *Diagnostic and Statistical Manual of Mental Disorders* (5th ed.; DSM-5). According to Dr. Robert D. Hare, one of the foremost experts on psychopaths and the developer of the most widely used assessment instrument in the identification of a psychopathy (PCL; Hare 1991), psychopaths tend to be callous, remorseless, and lacking in empathy. They are glib and superficial, manipulative, impulsive, and antisocial (Hare & Neumann, 2008). It is estimated that 1% of the general male population are psychopaths; however, these percentages increase based on contextual factors. For example, approximately 15–20% of the prison population meet Hare's criteria for psychopathy (Häkkänen-Nyholm & Hare, 2009). Psychopaths pose a real threat to society and are often found within the criminal justice system. However, this does not mean that all individuals with psychopathic traits are criminals. More recent literature indicates that psychopathic traits can exist on a continuum, and individuals with psychopathic traits may not necessarily exhibit the same severity of symptoms (Skeem, Polaschek, Patrick & Lilienfeld, 2011). Furthermore, just because an individual meets the generally accepted threshold for psychopathy does not mean they will exhibit criminal behaviors. These considerations have incited debate in recent literature regarding the inclusion of criminality in the factorial structure of psychopathy. Some experts argue for a two-, three-, or four-factor model of psychopathy (Skeem & Cooke, 2010). By removing criminal behavior as a key component for psychopathy, researchers can examine psychopathic traits within a general population. These individuals are found in all areas of society and regularly lead successful lives.

Current evidence suggests that psychopathy is a lifelong disorder and has a biological basis. A combination of genetic and environmental influences contributes to these traits and their manifestations in an individual (MacDonald & Iacono, 2006). Characteristics may be identified early in childhood, particularly callous-unemotional traits. It is important to understand theories and development when attempting to recognize psychopaths. Hare's Psychopathy Checklist-Revised (PCL-R; Hare) is the most used psychological assessment in the identification of psychopathic individuals. It has 20 items and utilizes a semi-structured interview to produce scores on a three-point scale. Out of a maximum score of 40, the label of psychopathy is usually given to those who score above 30. There are many uses of this assessment and versions, including a screening version and a youth version. Although the PCL-R should only be administered by an experienced clinician, understanding the traits identified in the assessment is helpful in recognizing a psychopath.

The primary aim of this brief is to further explore the research on psychopaths in different settings and everyday life. Psychopaths are often predatory by nature but may appear normal to laypersons. Individuals who work in health professions, forensic occupations, education, and corporate environments are likely to encounter someone with psychopathic traits at some point in their careers. Psychopaths have little difficulty blending into everyday situations. When working in a setting where one might encounter an individual with psychopathic characteristics – whether that person is a colleague, client, supervisor, or boss – it is important to be able to identify them, understand the implications, and navigate any necessary interactions.

Fort Lauderdale, FL, USA   Tom D. Kennedy
                                                                                               Elise Anello
                                                                                       Stephanie Sardinas
                                                                                     Scarlet Paria Woods

References

American Psychiatric Association. (2013). *Diagnostic and statistical manual of mental disorders* (5th ed.). https://doi.org/10.1176/appi.books.9780890425596.

Häkkänen-Nyholm, H., & Hare, R. D. (2009). Psychopathy, homicide, and the courts: Working the system. *Criminal Justice and Behavior, 36*(8), 761–777. https://doi.org/10.1177/0093854809336946.

Hare, R. D., & Neumann, C. S. (2008). Psychopathy as a clinical and empirical construct. *Annual Review of Clinical Psychology, 4*, 217–246. https://doi.org/10.1146/annurev.clinpsy.3.022806.09145.

Hare, R. D. (1991). *The hare psychopathy checklist-revised*. Multi-Health Systems.

MacDonald, A. W. III, & Iacono, W. G. (2006). Toward an Integrated Perspective on the Etiology of Psychopathy. In C. J. Patrick (Ed.), *Handbook of psychopathy*. The Guilford Press, pp. 375–385.

Skeem, J. L., & Cooke, D. J. (2010). Is criminal behavior a central component of psychopathy? Conceptual directions for resolving the debate. *Psychological Assessment, 22*(2), 433–445. https://doi.org/10.1037/a0008512.

Skeem, J. L., Polaschek, D. L. L., Patrick, C. J., & Lilienfeld, S. O. (2011). Psychopathic personality: Bridging the gap between scientific evidence and public policy. *Psychological Science in the Public Interest, 12*(3), 95–162. https://doi.org/10.1177/1529100611426706

Contents

Chapter 1
Introduction to Psychopathy

1.1 What Is Psychopathy?

Philippe Pinel (1806/1962) may have first introduced the idea of what would become our modern-day understanding of psychopathy, which he labeled *manie sans delire* (insanity without delirium). He described an individual who did not suffer from any apparent clouding of the mind but was prone to dramatic episodes of impulsivity, recklessness, and aggression. A half century later, Julius Koch (1888) introduced the disease-oriented term "psychopathic" to convey the idea that the condition had a strong heritable basis, recently supported by twin and family studies. From these theoretical and anecdotal beginnings, a more empirical based examination of the construct was instigated by Cleckley. Cleckley (1941) in his seminal book *Mask of Sanity* further elaborated the psychopathic construct, describing an individual with superficial charm, lack of remorse, insincerity, lack of insight, and fantastic and objectionable behavior. Since then, an ever-growing body of research has deepened our understanding of psychopathy.

Hare (1985) further refined and operationalized the nature of a psychopath, characterized by glib and superficial charm, grandiose self-worth, pathological lying, manipulative style, lack of empathy, and parasitic lifestyle (freeloader), leading to his development of the Psychopathy Checklist (PCL). The purpose of the PCL was to identify individuals who met the criteria to be classified as a psychopath using a cutoff score (30 out of 40). Thus, a taxonic structure was assumed, meaning psychopaths were conceptualized as qualitatively distinct from non-psychopaths, rather than being characterized by extreme scores on a psychopathic personality continuum.

While the idea of psychopathy as a taxon has led to much controversy over the years, the PCL was a superb instrument having a profound impact on the field. The PCL was both parsimoniously and exhaustively constructed from a behavioral standpoint, encompassing most of the known behaviors of a psychopath at the time. As an aside, the taxon versus continuum dispute is not confined to researchers in the

T. D. Kennedy et al., *Working with Psychopathy*, SpringerBriefs in Psychology, https://doi.org/10.1007/978-3-030-84025-9_1

field of psychopathy, this debate is ongoing for most of the disorders classified in the Diagnostic and Statistical Manual of Mental Disorders (DSM-5). In fact, the consideration of mental disorders as a categorical entity (taxon) versus an extreme expression of continuously distributed traits is one of the longest standing debates among psychologists. Although a few diagnostic entities, like schizophrenia (Golden & Meehl, 1979), may be distributed as a discrete latent class, representing a typological difference from normal personality, psychopathy appears to represent more of a quantitative shift in normal personality.

Briefly, Meehl and colleagues provided a framework for taxometric analysis, providing 13 interconnected procedures (Meehl, 1999; Meehl & Yonce, 1994; Waller & Meehl, 1998). These procedures were developed to find abrupt changes (e.g., slopes, covariances) in the structure of the data, which would indicate a tax-onic structure or latent subgroups in a distribution of scores. These abrupt changes are not adequately supported from the taxometric analyses of psychopathy (Sellbom & Drislane, 2020).

1.2   Why Are There Psychopaths?

There is abundant literature providing various descriptions of psychopathy, but why are there psychopaths? Although the answer is not the premise for this brief, it is important to touch on some of the theory related to why psychopaths exist in society today. Before we address the more specific occupational based adaptive and mal-adaptive characteristics associated with psychopathy, a short exploration of the "ultimate explanation" for the existence of psychopathy is warranted. Understanding the ultimate explanation or evolved function of a behavior or trait is the main aim of evolutionary psychologists. Could it be that the traits associated with psychopathy are adaptive? This idea may seem paradoxical, since from an evolutionary perspec-tive, much of our social behavior is grounded in acts of reciprocation and coopera-tion (Trivers, 1985). In fact, there is a large body of work in the field of evolutionary game theory that supports the emergence and stability of cooperation and reciproca-tion as critical for our survival. So why did the parasitic nature of psychopaths sur-vive throughout the course of our evolution as a species?

It is possible that a small subset of individuals exhibiting parasitic characteristics emerged within the larger cooperative, reciprocation-based societal structure. This small subset of individuals (non-reciprocators) may have adapted to benefit in dif-ferent ways from most individuals whose behaviors are based more on cooperation (Trivers, 1985). In other words, perhaps these non-reciprocating individuals learned how to "beat" the system, to take advantage of their naïve reciprocating counter-parts. These freeloaders, as evolutionists sometimes refer to them, may have stum-bled on an effective alternative adaptive strategy or a life history strategy with some traits even aiding reproductive survival success (Mealey, 1995).

Evolutionists like Mealey (2005a, b) explicitly refer to the non-reciprocation nature of psychopaths, while McGuire and Troisi (1998) explicate this non-reciprocation idea to antisocial personality disorder (ASPD), a disorder that substantially overlaps psychopathy. For this idea to hold true, there are two general premises that evolutionists consider key to the long-term survival (existence and maintenance) of psychopaths in society. First, psychopathy would require genetic underpinnings, and second, psychopaths should only make up a small percentage (i.e., rare type) of the population. If the balance shifts and the percentage of the population of psychopaths expands, the system will break down. This is known as frequency-dependent selection, meaning the fitness of a given genotype depends on its frequency (Frank, 1988; Mealey, 1995). Psychopaths do in fact represent a rare type, indicating a negative frequency dependence. One-sided frequency dependence occurs when the advantage holds only for one type when rare. In this case, the rare type (psychopath) may have a unique competitive advantage compared to the common type (cooperative) when the ratio is balanced, but when the rarer type becomes more common, the advantage vanishes (as the psychopaths are exposed) and the percentage of non-reciprocating psychopaths in the population drops. Perhaps homeostasis is maintained through a continually naturally balancing between the rare and common type, keeping the current estimates of psychopaths somewhere around 1% of the population.

There is considerable evidence for these two premises. The genetic premise is supported by brain science as well as twin and family studies (Levenston et al., 2000; Patrick et al., 1994; Raine et al., 2004; Schulsinger, 1972), while the small percentage of psychopaths in the general population supports the second premise. Additional investigations utilizing neuroimaging to explore the biological basis of psychopathy provide further evidence for a highly heritable disorder (Blonigen et al., 2005). Researchers detected decreased gray matter volume (GMV) in the limbic (Contreras-Rodríguez, 2014; Ermer et al., 2012; Yang et al., 2010) and frontotemporal areas of the brain (Yang et al., 2010). Defects in the default mode network also exist (Anderson et al., 2018; Greicius et al., 2003). Further dysfunction was also found in areas of the brain (mesolimbic and paralimbic) associated with empathy (Diamond & Dickenson, 2012).

As an aside, the disproportionate number of male psychopaths may be explained by the (a) cheater hypothesis, (b) warrior-hawk hypothesis, and the (c) cheater-hawk hypothesis. Evolutionarily speaking, a cheater represents someone who is uncooperative or cooperates less than others and takes more than their fair share of collective resources to maximize their own individual fitness (Ferriere et al., 2002; West et al., 2006). The cheater hypothesis may be adaptive (Mealey, 1995) when the benefits of cheating outweigh the costs and when the cheaters are the rare type (fewer cheaters than cooperators). Cheaters are less likely to be caught if they move from group to group (i.e., to different geographically areas); this type of movement is known to have occurred disproportionality in males who evolved with greater migratory tendencies. Evolutionists also suggest that men may have needed to compete more than women, especially when it came to finding a mate, and thus were more likely to exhibit duplicitous behavior to win in mating competition.

Although the cheater hypothesis, which provides a framework for increased duplicity and manipulation, may offer some clue to why male psychopaths outnumber females, it provides no explanation for the aggressive component of psychopathy. The warrior-hawk hypothesis addresses this aspect and accounts for both the psychopath's reactivity to slights and their use of intimidation, and both are characteristics more highly associated with males. Finally, the cheater-hawk hypothesis reflects a combination of both theories, cheater (short-term mating orientation) and hawk (aggression). Researchers found a strong relationship between the cheater-hawk theory and psychopathy as psychopaths tend to use individualistic and competitive strategies in an altruism game (Book et al., 2019). A classic example of this is the "Prisoner's Dilemma" where an uncooperative strategy may be chosen even when cooperation may be the best choice. Types of short-term uncooperative mating strategies and aggressive behaviors are more prevalent in males (Buss & Schmitt, 2019) which may help to explain the higher proportion of male psychopaths. Furthermore, as selection favored stronger migratory tendency in males, perhaps male psychopaths were less likely to be exposed as they moved more frequently between groups.

Some evolutionists propose different subgroups of psychopathy, which is particularly relevant to the current brief. Perhaps Karpman (1941) was the first to present the idea of ecological structures that differentiate between types of criminal psychopaths. One group, he termed "primary psychopathy," includes individuals born with a certain predisposition hindering their development of a conscious (lack of guilt and empathy), while the other group (secondary psychopathy) were more aggressive and impulsive, and although may have some genetic predisposition, their conscience formation was more impacted by environmental factors (Karpman, 1941). Thus, the term sociopathy is fairly consistent with the secondary psychopathic conceptualization, implying that the antisocial tendencies are primarily the result of environmental factors like poor socialization rather than genetic underpinnings (Lykken, 1995). This distinction between psychopathy (primary) and sociopathy (secondary) is consistent with more current findings which indicate a greater history of abuse and maltreatment among the secondary type (Blackburn et al., 2008; Kimonis et al., 2012) versus the nonshared environmental influences of the primary type (Viding et al., 2008, Vernon et al., 2008). Mealey (1995), from an evolutionary perspective, also considered these two subgroups as primary and secondary psychopaths.

1.3   Primary Versus Secondary Psychopathy

Karpman (1941), with his specification of a primary and secondary type, was very influential on the course of study in the field of psychopathy. Although there was much overlap between the types, clear etiological and motivational differences distinguished the two. The primary type was considered heritable as these individuals were born without a conscience, while the secondary type was manifested through psychosocial learning by some type of trauma, abuse, or parental rejection (Karpman, 1941). Furthermore, Karpman considered the primary type as treatment resistant (incurable), while the secondary type could be helped through therapy as the origins are more environmental in nature, and moral and ethical reasoning was only clouded through the conflict they endured. Many of the differentiations between psychopaths and sociopaths noted in Table 1.1 seem to parallel Karpman's original idea of primary versus secondary psychopathy. In fact, we would argue that the historical idea of primary versus secondary psychopathy is synonymous with the more recent psychopathy versus sociopathy distinction.

Years later, Mealey (1995) further explored the types of psychopathy first introduced by Karpman, with a focus on the age-old nature versus nurture debate. According to Mealey (1995), primary psychopaths have a genetic mechanism for maintaining their adaptive cheating strategies, so their numbers remain relatively

Table 1.1 Discriminators between psychopathy and sociopathy found in the literature

Psychopath	Sociopath
Strong heritable contributions (greater genetic predisposition)	Gene-environment interactions
*Lack of empathy and guilt (no conscience)	Sense of morality and potential well-developed conscience
Asymmetry with antisocial personality disorder	More overlap with antisocial personality disorder
Less inclined to crime	More inclined to crime
*Unemotional	Emotional
*Does not feel remorse	Feels remorse usually with the group they identify with only
*Cold, calculated, logical	Violent, erratic, rational
*Higher IQ	Lower IQ
*Patient	Impatient
*Likely to be educated and have a good career	Likely to be uneducated and not be able to keep a steady job
*Highly manipulative, less impulsive	Impulsive, spontaneous
*Unable to form personal attachments (does not bond with anyone)	May form attachments with an individual or group (bonds with primary group)
Nonshared environmental influences	Likely to have experienced childhood trauma or abuse (shared environmental influences)
*More planning in acting out	Risk taking, impulsive
*Able to hide deprecating attitude	Not able to hide deprecating attitude
Reduced fear, anxiety, and shock avoidance	Higher on fear, anxiety, and shock avoidance scales
*No IQ imbalance	IQ imbalance with performance being higher than verbal
Stable trait with a constant prevalence across time, culture, and socioeconomic status	Fluctuates with changes in sociocultural environments
Approximately 3–15% of antisocial personality disorder cases	Approximately 30% of antisocial personality disorder cases
Not likely to be easily angered	Prone to anger and violent outbursts

*Germane to this brief

stable compared to the secondary psychopaths, who exhibit a more environmentally based mechanism for maintaining their cheating strategy. Although there is considerable debate regarding these subgroups, there is some support for the idea that primary psychopathy is more innate with greater genetically based factors compared to secondary psychopathy, which is viewed more as adaptation to environmental risk (based largely on life experiences and environmental contingencies).

According to Mealey (1995), primary psychopaths are born, not made, while secondary psychopaths are a product of an interaction between a genetic predisposition and specific environmental factors. While the characteristics of the primary psychopath may be specified by their genes, the secondary type inherits only a predisposition to adopt the freeloading or parasitic lifestyle discussed earlier. Thus, for the secondary type, the emergence of a psychopathic personality is dependent upon the environment where the individual is raised and may be more likely to manifest when the individual is competitively disadvantaged to obtain resources. Individuals with this type may be more likely develop in an environment with a dense population where cheating is less likely to be exposed and there are more opportunities to do so, or in environments where cooperation does not improve one's access to resources.

1.4 Psychopathy, Sociopathy, and Antisocial Personality Disorder (ASPD)

Although there is no psychopathy diagnosis in the DSM-5, it briefly mentions psychopathy, sociopathy, and dissocial personality disorder (the antisocial personality disorder equivalent from the International Classification of Diseases, ICD-10) as terms that represent a pervasive pattern of disregard for, and violation of, the rights of others (essential feature of ASPD). More specifically, the ASPD section of the DSM-5 specifies a "lack of empathy, inflated self-appraisal, and superficial charm are features that have been commonly included in traditional conceptions of psychopathy." While no formal diagnosis exists, there is abundant research and clinical evidence, as well as multiple assessments focused on the construct of psychopathy. For clarity, a brief discussion differentiating APSD, psychopathy, and sociopathy is warranted.

The terms psychopathy, sociopathy, and ASPD are often associated with a similar constellation of traits found to varying degrees in each. However, a growing consensus supports the distinction between psychopathy and sociopathy, each having their own unique etiology and motivational drivers, with the clinical diagnosis of ASPD being applicable to both (Walsh & Wu, 2008). In fact, there is an increasing number of researchers attempting to operationalize these terms for clarity and specificity. Although clarifying these three concepts as separate and distinct is helpful for research purposes, the borders separating them are more likely porous and fuzzy with many overlapping characteristics. For clarity and for the purpose of this brief, we will operationalize each before setting our focus on psychopathy for the remainder of the chapters.

Of the three terms, the DSM-5 only offers a diagnosis for ASPD and suggests a prevalence rate of about 3% for males and 1% for females (American Psychiatric Association 2013; Marten, 2000). Interestingly, approximately 3–15% of those with ASPD also exhibit psychopathy and an additional 30% sociopathy (Johnson, 2019). The overlapping nature of the three constructs may imply that sociopathy and psychopathy are extreme forms of ASPD. To further complicate the matter, the terms sociopath and psychopath are often used interchangeably, and both essentially meet the diagnostic criteria for ASPD; however, there is support for two distinct constructs. Although both include many of the same associated behaviors and characteristics, the etiology of psychopathy is often considered more neurological while sociopathy more environmental. There is a growing consensus that provides some clarity between the sociopath and the psychopath. The stability and prevalence of psychopaths across time and across class lines support the biological bases. Although the DSM-5 seems to conceptualize the three constructs as roughly the same, ignoring the differential nuances may limit both a clinician's ability to provide optimal services and a researcher's desire for clearly operationalized constructs.

Again, a distinguishing characteristic of psychopathy is that the percentage of psychopaths across class lines remains remarkably stable over time. Although the data are not unequivocal, there is evidence that the origin of psychopathy is not primarily developmental or sociocultural in nature (Pitchford, 2001). In fact, there is an expanding body of evidence (Blonigen et al., 2005; Brook et al., 2010; Larsson et al., 2006; Vernon et al., 2008) for a genetic basis which supports Hare's (1993) earlier assertions that social or environmental factors were not the root cause of psychopathy. An important caveat to many of the studies which explore this aspect of psychopathy is that some authors have considered ASPD and psychopathy synonymous. Hare (1993) and others cautioned against this; although there is evidence for much overlap between ASPD and psychopathy, there is clear asymmetry. This asymmetry is evident when comparing PCL scores. While almost all PCL psychopaths meet criteria for ASPD, only a small percentage of individuals with ASPD meet criteria for psychopathy (Hare, 1996).

Rhee and Waldman (2002) provide further support for the strong genetic component of psychopathy. The authors in this case were careful to acknowledge the threat of considering ASPD tantamount to psychopathy and thus ran two analyses, one with the ASPD samples alone and one with the inclusion of eight samples of psychopathy. Interestingly, the inclusion of the eight psychopathic specific samples did not alter the results of the meta-analysis. The model including (a) additive genetic influences, (b) shared environmental influences, (c) nonadditive genetic influences, and (d) nonshared environmental influences with data from all the twin and adoption studies indicated additive genetic (the effect of multiple genes that exert influence in a linear or additive fashion) and nonshared environmental influences and very little evidence for shared environmental effects (which is more associated with sociopathy). Not only does this data support a strong genetic component of psychopathy, it reinforces Hare's (1993) assertion that psychopathy is not caused by shared environmental influences, but rather genetics and individual-specific environmental effects. This is noteworthy as there is ample evidence for shared environmental contributions to ASPD. Perhaps this evidence supports the notion that ASPD and sociopathy describe a broader, more behavioral based biologically heterogenous group than psychopathy. This differentiation provides a good point of departure from psychopathy to the related construct of sociopathy.

While the root of psychopathy may tend toward the nature side of the nature/nurture continuum, sociopathy origins are usually considered more nurture based. In fact, Mealey (1995) intimated that the cheating strategy of the sociopath may be less connected to the genotype than it is with the psychopath, while Lykken (1995) theorized that sociopathy develops through an interaction between deviant learning histories and deviant genetic predilections. Unlike the case of a psychopath (nonshared environmental influences), the learning history is more of the shared type (e.g., hostile childhood experiences). Hare and Babiek (2006) provided more clarification regarding how sociopathy differs from psychopathy. A sociopath has a sense of morality and a well-developed conscious; however, their sense of right and wrong is not aligned with the cultural and societal mores (Hare & Babiek, 2006). Lykken (1995) perceives the threat of sociopaths (in terms of damage to society) as more concerning than the threat of psychopaths, as they are equally as dangerous but more numerous.

1.5   Nature of Psychopathy

Much of our understanding of the nature of psychopathy comes from the PCL and PCL-R (Hare, 1991, 2003). Having a single instrument shape so much of our understanding of psychopathy may have led to some of the complex challenge's researchers in the field of psychopathy face today. There are even some who have expressed concerns that the instrument became the construct (Cooke et al., 2005); however there has been clear expansion, exploration, and testing of multiple theories and measurement tools over the past decades. The factor structure and even the conceptualization of psychopathy continue to be debated among and between clinicians and researchers. Perhaps a bit frustratingly, the following sentiment of the nature of psychopathy still rings true today:

> Currently, there is little agreement on the most appropriate operational criteria for clinical diagnosis or for research. Indeed, the various clinical-behavioral and self-report procedures in common use differ widely in reliability and validity and clearly are not interchangeable with one another (Hare, 1985). As a result, there is no assurance that different investigators—all ostensibly engaged in research on psychopathy—are in fact dealing with the same disorder (Harpur et al., 1989, p. 6).

Although the two primary factors most associated with psychopathy (personality traits and antisocial behaviors) demonstrate differential relationships, there is still some support for a unidimensional structure as measured by the PCL (Harpur et al., 1989). However, the authors seem to lean toward the former conceptualization concluding that psychopathy need not be conceptualized as a unidimensional construct representing some endpoint of a dimension of normal personality, but rather its emergence may come from the interaction of certain personality characteristics and exposure to specific developmental influences (Harpur et al., 1989). Sellbom and Drislane (2020) echo this sentiment claiming that psychopathy is not unitary and suggest that all available research support their claim of a multidimensional construct. The authors discuss the nature of psychopathy consisting of multiple constellations of characteristics held together by an overarching factor (Sellbom & Drislane, 2020). These ideas not only suggest a complex manifestation of psychopathy through various personality and behavioral tendencies influenced by the environment but also bring into question the idea that psychopathy is a taxonic construct established by some threshold score. Although not yet a consensus, as can be seen in earlier work that endorsed taxometric properties (Harris et al., 1994), most recent studies provide substantial evidence for a dimensional structure rather than a latent taxon, with high and low scores on the PCL and PCL-R indicating differences in degree rather than qualitative differences in kind (Edens, et al., 2006; Edens, et al., 2011; Marcus, et al., 2004; Sellbom & Drislane, 2020; Walters, et al., 2007, 2015).

1.6   Factor Structure

Patrick (2006) and Hare and Newman (2005) discuss the variations of four constructs that continue to be most often cited at the core of psychopathy as interpersonal characteristics (e.g., superficial charm, grandiosity, deceitful, manipulative), affective traits (e.g., lack of empathy and remorse, shallow), impulsivity (e.g., irresponsible, parasitic lifestyle), and antisocial tendencies (e.g., poor behavioral control, criminal versatility). We will discuss the two-factor, three-factor, four-factor, LSRP, PPI, EPA (psychopathy from perspective of FFM), and triarchic model (boldness, meanness, and disinhibition) of psychopathy in more detail in the next chapter. However, the conceptualization of psychopathy as it relates to criminality or antisocial behavior warrants a brief discussion to clarify before moving forward. The debate over whether antisocial tendencies are a necessary component of psychopathy may have its roots in Cleckley's original conceptualization. Cleckley intimated a type of psychopath who displayed the core features of psychopathy; however, was never incarcerated. This could mean that this type of psychopath either (a) exhibited antisocial behaviors but committed no crimes, (b) broke the law but evaded incarceration, or (c) displayed elements of the interpersonal, affective, and impulsivity traits but lacked the antisocial tendencies. Or perhaps they possessed different combinations of the above. This has led to ongoing debate, research, and development of different factor models, with and without the antisocial features. To better understand this distinction, the need to examine the nature of psychopathy in community samples has been long theorized (Widom, 1977) and more recently empirically explored (Eisenbarth & Centifanti, 2020; Falkenbach et al., 2014; Neumann & Hare, 2008).

1.7   Successful Psychopaths

Psychopaths who evade criminal conviction or who abstain from criminal behavior are often deemed "successful" psychopaths. To be clear, success in this sense does not imply that these individuals are successful in other areas of their lives (Yang et al., 2010). However, the nature of successful versus unsuccessful psychopaths is particularly relevant to this brief. More specifically, the idea of a successful psychopath has garnered increasing interest from researchers in recent years. As discussed earlier, there is evidence that psychopathy is a dimensional rather than taxonic construct. Meaning there may be a continuum of psychopathic traits and perhaps where one falls on this continuum, in terms of severity and amount, along with how these traits interact with one's environment and upbringing may lead to a more or less successful manifestation. Lilienfeld and his colleagues (2014) found intriguing evidence for a link between adaptive attributes associated with various careers (e.g., high risk jobs, leadership, and management positions) and various psychopathic traits (e.g., social and physical boldness). Others have found similar relationships in other life areas (Benning et al., 2018; Blickle & Genau, 2019; Patton et al., 2018; Schütte et al., 2016; Titze et al., 2017) indicating that some characteristics of psychopathy may be adaptive in a wide range of work and life domains.

Unsuccessful psychopaths (unlike successful ones) have some distinct differences in their brain (Yang et al., 2005; Yang et al., 2009), psychophysiology (Gao et al., 2010; Ishikawa, et al. 2001), and cognition (Ishikawa et al., 2001; Mahmut et al., 2008). These differences represent (a) reduced volumes in the prefrontal cortex and the amygdala, (b) abnormalities in the hippocampus, and (c) deficits in executive function. Deficiencies in these areas may provide some clues to why some psychopaths are less successful than others. More specifically, deficits in these areas are known correlates of antisocial behavior and impulsivity which are more associated with sociopaths or secondary psychopaths who are more inclined to crime, less able to hold down a steady job, and more violent and erratic. This is in stark contrast to successful psychopaths, who demonstrate no (a) structural and functional defects in their prefrontal cortex, amygdala, or hippocampus (Yang, et al. 2005); (b) information processing dysfunction (Gao et al. 2011); (c) abnormalities in their autonomic nervous system (Ishikawa et al., 2001); and (d) deficits in executive functioning (Ishikawa et al., 2001). There is even some evidence for enhanced executive functioning, cognitive controls, and higher levels of intelligence (Baskin-Sommers et al., 2015; Ishikawa et al., 2001; Wall et al., 2013) among successful psychopaths. Perhaps, as Babiak and Hare (2006) intimated, primary psychopaths can use some of the interpersonal traits, along with these enhancements in executive function, in an adaptive way to procure status and resources with minimal effort and maximum gain (freeloaders) while downregulating their antisocial tendencies.

There is more evidence to support the idea of a successful psychopath, going all the way back to Cleckley (1941) who provided some support that was more theoretical in nature. Originally, Cleckley (1941) included some adaptive aspects to his conceptualization of psychopathy, with social potency, low anxiety, and stress immunity, while more recently others have introduced fearlessness (Lilienfeld et al., 2015; Lykken, 1995; Patton et al., 2018). There is also some preliminary evidence that successful psychopaths have low levels of agreeableness and higher levels of conscientiousness, self-discipline, and boldness (Lilienfeld et al., 2015, Mullins-Sweat et al., 2010). Further, Benning and his colleagues (2003) found that the fearless and socially dominant traits were positively correlated with educational attainment and resilience against internalizing disorders. These adaptive traits of executive functioning, autonomic responsivity, conscientiousness, boldness, and intelligence, along with others like social poise and superficial charm (Lilienfeld et al. 2016; Patton et al., 2018), may either serve to buffer against some of the more maladaptive antisocial tendencies, or they may work in tandem with traits that are generally considered maladaptive like lack of empathy and guilt, along with deceit and manipulation to help individuals succeed in certain careers discussed throughout this brief. When you couple the adaptive and maladaptive traits associated with psychopathy with their interaction with external variables like positive childhood experiences (Frick & White, 2008; Waller et al., 2013), you have the bases for the moderated-expression model proposed by Lilienfeld and his colleagues (2015). This model provides a unified foundation for the construct of a successful psychopath by subsuming the more recently considered adaptive traits along with the traditional core psychopathic traits and the interaction between external variables and these psychopathic characteristics.

References

American Psychiatric Association. (2013). *Diagnostic and statistical manual of mental disorders* (5th ed.).

Anderson, N. E., Maurer, J. M., Steele, V. R., & Kiehl, K. A. (2018). Psychopathic traits associated with abnormal hemodynamic activity in salience and default mode networks during auditory oddball task. *Cognitive, Affective, & Behavioral Neuroscience, 18*(3), 564–580.

Babiak, P., & Hare, R. D. (2006). *Snakes in suits: When psychopaths go to work*. Regan Books/Harper Collins Publishers.

Baskin-Sommers, A. R., Waller, R., Fish, A. M., & Hyde, L. W. (2015). Callous-Unemotional traits trajectories interact with earlier conduct problems and executive control to predict violence and substance use among high risk male adolescents. *Journal of Abnormal Child Psychology, 43*(8), 1529–1541.

Benning, S. D., Patrick, C. J., Hicks, B. M., Blonigen, D. M., & Krueger, R. F. (2003). Factor structure of the psychopathic personality inventory: Validity and implications for clinical assessment. *Psychological Assessment, 15*, 340–350.

Benning, S. D., Dowgwillo, E. A., & Miller, K. F. (2018). Psychopathy in the medical emergency department. *Journal of Personality Disorders, 32*(4), 482–496.

Blackburn, R., Logan, C., Donnelly, J. P., & Renwick, S. J. (2008). Identifying psychopathic subtypes: Combining an empirical personality classification of offenders with the Psychopathy Checklist-Revised. *Journal of Personality Disorders, 22*(6), 604–622.

Blickle, G., & Genau, H. A. (2019). The two faces of fearless dominance and their relations to vocational success. *Journal of Research in Personality, 81*, 25–37.

Blonigen, D. M., Hicks, B. M., Kruger, R. F., Patrick, C. J., & Iacono, W. G. (2005). Psychopathic personality traits: Heritability and genetic overlap with internalizing and externalizing psychopathology. *Psychological Medicine, 35*(5), 637–648.

Book, A., Methot-Jones, T., Blais, J., Hosker-Field, A., Volk, A., Visser, B. A., Gauthier, N., Holden, R. R., & D'Agata, M. T. (2019). Psychopathic traits and the cheater-hawk hypothesis. *Journal of Interpersonal Violence, 34*(15), 3229–3251.

Brook, M., Panizzon, M., Kosson, D., Sullivan, E. A., Lyons, M., Franz, C., Eisen, S., & Kremen, W. (2010). Psychopathic personality traits in middle-aged male twins: a behavior genetic investigation. *Journal of Personality Disorders, 24*(4), 473–486.

Buss, D. M., & Schmitt, D. P. (2019). Mate Preferences and Their Behavioral Manifestations. *Annual Review of Psychology, 70*, 77–110.

Cleckley, H. (1941). *The mask of sanity; an attempt to reinterpret the so-called psychopathic personality*. Mosby.

Contreras-Rodríguez, O., Pujol, J., Batalla, I., Harrison, B. J., Bosque, J., Ibern-Regàs, I., et al. (2014). Disrupted neural processing of emotional faces in psychopathy. *Social Cognitive and Affective Neuroscience, 9*(4), 505–512.

Cooke, D. J., Michie, C., Hart, S. D., & Clark, D. (2005). Searching for the pan-cultural core of psychopathic personality disorder. *Personality and Individual Differences, 39*, 283–295.

Diamond, L. M., & Dickenson, J. A. (2012). The neuroimaging of love and desire: Review and future directions. *Clinical Neuropsychiatry, 9*(1), 39–46.

Edens, J. F., Marcus, D. K., Lilienfeld, S. O., & Poythress, N. G., Jr. (2006). Psychopathic, not psychopath: Taxometric evidence for the dimensional structure of psychopathy. *Journal of Abnormal Psychology, 115*(1), 131–144.

Edens, J. F., Marcus, D. K., & Vaughn, M. G. (2011). Exploring the taxometric status of psychopathy among youthful offenders: Is there a juvenile psychopath taxon? *Law and Human Behavior, 35*(1), 13–24.

Eisenbarth, H., & Centifanti, L. C. M. (2020). Dimensions of psychopathic traits in a community sample: Implications from different measures for impulsivity and delinquency. *European Journal of Psychological Assessment, 36*(1), 1–11.

Ermer, E., Cope, L. M., Nyalakanti, P. K., Calhoun, V. D., & Kiehl, K. A. (2012). Aberrant paralimbic gray matter in criminal psychopathy. *Journal of Abnormal Psychology, 121*(3), 649–658.

Falkenbach, D. M., Stern, S. B., & Creevy, C. (2014). Psychopathy variants: Empirical evidence supporting a subtyping model in a community sample. *Personality Disorders, Theory, Research, and Treatment, 5*(1), 10–19.

Ferriere, R., Bronstein, J. L., Rinaldi, S., Law, R., & Gauduchon, M. (2002). Cheating and the evolutionary stability of mutualisms. *Proceedings of the Biological Sciences, 269*(1493), 773–780.

Frank, R. H. (1988). *Passions with reason: the strategic role of the emotions*. W.W. Norton & Company.

Frick, P. J., & White, S. F. (2008). Research review: the importance of callous-unemotional traits for developmental models of aggressive and antisocial behavior. *Journal of Child Psychology and Psychiatry, 49*(4), 359–375.

Gao, Y., Raine, A., Yaralian, P., & Yang, Y. (2010). Somatic aphasia: Mismatch of body sensations with autonomic stress reactivity in psychopathy. *Biological Psychology, 90*, 228–233.

Gao, Y., Raine, A., & Schug, R. A. (2011). P3 event-related potentials and childhood maltreatment in successful and unsuccessful psychopaths. *Brain and Cognition, 77*(2), 176–182.

Golden, R. R., & Meehl, P. E. (1979). Detection of the schizoid taxon with MMPI indicators. *Journal of Abnormal Psychology, 88*, 217–233.

Greicius, M. D., Krasnow, B., Reiss, A. L., & Menon, V. (2003). Functional connectivity in the resting brain: A network analysis of the default mode hypothesis. *Proceedings of the National Academy of Sciences, 100*(1), 253–258.

Hare, R. D. (1985). Comparison of the procedures for the assessment of psychopathy. *Journal of Consulting and Clinical Psychology, 53*, 1–16.

Hare, R.D. (1991). The Hare Psychopathy Checklist – Revised. Multi Health Systems.

Hare, R. D. (1993). *Without conscience: The disturbing world of the psychopaths among us.* Pocket Books.

Hare, R. D. (1996). Psychopathy: a clinical construct whose time has come. *Criminal Justice and Behavior, 23*(1), 25–54.

Hare, R. D. (2003). *The Hare Psychopathy Checklist – Revised* (2nd ed.) Multi-Health Systems.

Hare, R. D., & Babiek, P. (2006). *Snakes in suits.* Harper Collins.

Hare, R. D., & Neumann, C. S. (2005). The structure of psychopathy. *Current Psychiatry Reports, 7*(1), 1–32.

Harpur, T. J., Hare, R. D., & Hakstian, A. R. (1989). Two-factor conceptualization of psychopathy: Construct validity and assessment implications. *Psychological Assessment: A Journal of Consulting and Clinical Psychology, 1,* 6–17.

Harris, G. T., Rice, M. E., & Quinsey, V. L. (1994). Psychopathy as a taxon: Evidence that psychopaths are a discrete class. *Journal of Consulting and Clinical Psychology, 62*(2), 387–397.

Ishikawa, S. S., Raine, A., Lencz, T., Bihrle, S., & LaCasse, L. (2001). Autonomic stress reactivity and executive functions in successful and unsuccessful criminal psychopaths from the community. *Journal of Abnormal Psychology, 110,* 423–432.

Johnson, S. A. (2019). Understanding the violent personality: antisocial personality disorder, psychopathy, & sociopathy explored. *Forensic Research & Criminology International Journal, 7*(2), 76–88.

Karpman, B. (1941). On the need of separating psychopathy into two distinct clinical types: The symptomatic and the idiopathic. *Journal of Criminal Psychopathology, 3,* 112–137.

Kimonis, E. R., Frick, P. J., Cauffman, E., Goldweber, A., & Skeem, J. (2012). Primary and secondary variants of juvenile psychopathy differ in emotional processing. *Development and Psychopathology, 24*(3), 1091–1103.

Koch, J. L. A. (1888). Kurzgefasster Leitfaden der Psychiatrie mit besonderer Rucksichtnahme auf die Berdurfnisse der Studierenden, der praktischen Arzte und der Gerichtsarzte. Ravensburg: Dorn.

Larsson, H., Andershed, H., & Lichtenstein, P. (2006). A genetic factor explains most of the variation in the psychopathic personality. *Journal of Abnormal Psychology, 115*(2), 221–230.

Levenston, G., Patrick, C., Bradley, M., & Lang, P. (2000). The psychopath as observer: Emotion and attention in picture processing. *Journal of Cognitive Neuroscience, 10*(4), 525–535.

Lilienfeld, S. O., Latzman, R. D., Watts, A. L., Smith, S. F., & Dutton, K. (2014). Correlates of psychopathic personality traits in everyday life: Results from a large community survey. *Frontiers in Psychology, 5,* 1–11.

Lilienfeld, S. O., Smith, S. F., Sauvigne, K. C., Patrick, C. J., Drislane, L. E., Latzman, R. D., & Krueger, R. F. (2016). Is boldness relevant to psychopathic personality? Meta-analytic relations with non-Psychopathy Checklist-based measures of psychopathy. *Psychological Assessment, 28*(10), 1172.

Lilienfeld S. O., Watts A. L., Smith S. F. (2015). Successful psychopathy: A scientific status report. *Current Directions in Psychological Science, 24*(4), 298–303. https://doi.org/10.1177/0963721415580297.

Lykken, D. (1995). *The antisocial personalities.* Psychology Press.

Mahmut, M. K., Homewood, J., & Stevenson, R. J. (2008). The characteristics of non-criminals with high psychopathy traits: Are they similar to criminal psychopaths? *Journal of Research in Personality, 42*(3), 679–692.

Marcus, D. K., John, S. L., & Edens, J. F. (2004). A taxometric analysis of psychopathic personality. *Journal of Abnormal Psychology, 113*(4), 626–635.

Martens, W. H. J. (2000). Antisocial and Psychopathic Personality Disorders: Causes, course, and remission – A review article. *International Journal of Offender Therapy and Comparative Criminology, 44*(4), 406–430.

McGuire, M., & Troisi, A. (1998). *Darwinian Psychiatry.* Oxford University Press.

Mealey, L. (1995). The sociobiology of sociopathy: An integrated evolutionary model. *Behavioral and Brain Sciences, 18,* 523–599.

Mealey, L. (2005a). Evolutionary psychopathology and abnormal development. In R. L. Burgess & K. MacDonald (Eds.), *Evolutionary Perspectives on Human Development* (2nd ed., pp. 381–406). Sage.

Mealey, L. (2005b). The sociobiology of sociopathy: An integrated evolutionary model. *Behavioral and Brain Sciences, 18*, 523–599.

Meehl, P. E. (1999). Clarifications about taxometric method. *Applied and Preventive Psychology, 8*, 165–174.

Meehl, P. E., & Yonce, L. J. (1994). Taxometric analysis: I. Detecting taxonicity with two quantitative indicators using means above and below a sliding cut (MAMBAC procedure). *Psychological Reports, 74*, 1059–1274.

Mullins-Sweatt, S. N., Glover, N. G., Derefinko, K. J., Miller, J. D., & Widiger, T. A. (2010). The search for the successful psychopath. *Journal of Research in Personality, 44*(4), 554–558.

Neumann, C. S., & Hare, R. D. (2008). Psychopathic traits in a large community sample: Links to violence, alcohol use, and intelligence. *Journal of Consulting and Clinical Psychology, 76*(5), 893–899.

Patrick, C. J. (2006). *Back to the future: Cleckley as a guide to the next generation of psychopathy research*. In C. J. Patrick (Ed.), *Handbook of psychopathy*. Guilford Press.

Patrick, C., Cuthbert, B., & Lang, P. (1994). Emotion in the criminal psychopath: Fear image processing. *Journal of Abnormal Psychology, 103*(3), 519–528.

Patton, C. L., Smith, S. F., & Lilienfeld, S. O. (2018). Psychopathy and heroism in first responders: Traits cut from the same cloth? *Personality Disorders, Theory, Research, and Treatment, 9*(4), 354–368.

Pitchford, I. (2001). The origins of violence: Is psychopathy an adaptation? *Human Nature Review, 1*, 28–38.

Raine, A., Ishikawa, S., Arce, E., Lencz, T., & Colletti, P. (2004). Hippocampal structural asymmetry in unsuccessful psychopaths. *Biological Psychiatry, 55*, 185–191.

Rhee, S. H., & Waldman, I. D. (2002). Genetic and environmental influences on antisocial behavior: A meta-analysis of twin and adoption studies. *Psychological Bulletin, 128*(3), 490–529.

Schulsinger, F. (1972). Psychopathy, heredity and environment. *International Journal of Mental Health, 1*, 190–206.

Schütte, N., Blickle, G., Frieder, R. E., Wihler, A., Schnitzler, F., Heupel, J., & Zettler, I. (2016). The role of interpersonal influence in counterbalancing psychopathic personality trait facets at work. *Journal of Management, 44*(4), 1338–1368.

Sellbom, M., & Drislane, L. E. (2020). The classification of psychopathy. *Aggression and Violent Behavior, 101473*.

Titze, J. L., Blickle, G., & Wihler, A. (2017). Fearless dominance and performance in field sales: A predictive study. *International Journal of Selection and Assessment, 25*(3), 299–310.

Trivers, R. L. (1985). *Social Evolution*. Benjamins/Cummings.

Vernon, P. A., Villani, V. C., Vickers, L. C., & Harris, J. A. (2008). A behavioral genetic investigation of the Dark Triad and the Big 5. *Personality and Individual Differences, 44*(2), 445–452.

Viding, E., Jones, A. P., Frick, P. J., Moffitt, T. E., & Plomin, R. (2008). Heritability of antisocial behaviour at 9: Do callous-unemotional traits matter? *Developmental Science, 11*(1), 17–22.

Wall, T. D., Sellbom, M., & Goodwin, B. E. (2013). Examination of Intelligence as a Compensatory Factor in Non-Criminal Psychopathy in a Non-Incarcerated Sample. *Journal of Psychopathology and Behavioral Assessment, 35*(4), 450–459.

Waller, N. G., & Meehl, P. E. (1998). *Multivariate taxometric procedures: Distinguishing types from continua*. Sage.

Walsh, A., & Wu, H. (2008). Differentiating antisocial personality disorder, psychopathy, and sociopathy: Evolutionary, genetic, neurological, and sociological considerations. *Criminal Justice Studies: A Critical Journal of Crime, Law & Society, 21*(2), 135–152.

Walters, G. D., Duncan, S. A., & Mitchell-Perez, K. (2007). The latent structure of psychopathy: A taxometric investigation of the Psychopathy Checklist – Revised in a heterogeneous sample of male prison inmates. *Assessment, 14*(3), 270–278.

Walters, G. D., Ermer, E., Knight, R. A., & Kiehl, K. A. (2015). Paralimbic biomarkers in taxometric analyses of psychopathy: Does changing the indicators change the conclusion? *Personality Disorders, Theory, Research, and Treatment, 6*(1), 41–52.

West, S. A., Griffin, A. S., Gardner, A., & Diggle, S. P. (2006). Social evolution theory for microorganisms. *Nature Reviews Microbiology, 4*(8), 597–607.

Widom, C. S. (1977). A methodology for studying noninstitutionalized psychopaths. *Journal of Consulting and Clinical Psychology, 45,* 674–683.

Yang, Y., Raine, A., Lencz, T., Bihrle, S., LaCasse, L., & Colletti, P. (2005). Volume reduction in prefrontal gray matter in unsuccessful criminal psychopaths. *Biological Psychiatry, 57*(10), 1103–1108.

Yang, Y., Raine, A., Narr, K. L., Colletti, P., & Toga, A. W. (2009). Localization of deformations within the amygdala in individuals with psychopathy. *Archives of General Psychiatry, 66*(9), 986–994.

Yang, Y., Raine, A., Colletti, P., Toga, A. W., & Narr, K. L. (2010). Morphological alterations in the prefrontal cortex and the amygdala in unsuccessful psychopaths. *Journal of Abnormal Psychology, 119*(3), 546–554.

Chapter 2
Recognizing a Psychopath: Conceptual Confusion

This chapter is not meant to aid in diagnosis nor is it intended for use in professional decision-making. It is for informational and educational purposes only.

Despite over half a century of empirical research, considerable professional debate remains over the nature of the construct of psychopathy and how it is best measured. Depending on what conceptualization of psychopathy is referenced, the central focus of the construct differs (e.g., Lilienfeld et al., 2012; Widiger & Lynam, 1998). For instance, scholars have disagreed on whether the construct of psychopathy reflects qualitative deficits in neurobiology or personality or, rather, is comprised of a distinctive assemblage of general personality traits (e.g., Miller & Lynam, 2015). Scientifically speaking, this is a debate over the categorical (presence or lack of deficits, psychopathy or not) versus dimensional (to what *degree* are psychopathic traits present) quality of the construct. Steady across all conceptualizations is the belief that psychopathic individuals reflect a lower level of conscientiousness or concern for the rights of others that is displayed through varying degrees of socially unacceptable behavior. It is important to note that while there are decades of literature attempting to describe the construct of psychopathy, some of its features can be inherently challenging to distinguish and observe empirically. For instance, manipulation is considered a core feature of some psychopathy conceptualizations (e.g., Hare, 1991, 2003), yet the deceit that is enacted, by its very nature, can be difficult to identify.

To this day, researchers and clinicians have primarily relied on Hare's conceptualization of psychopathy, as measured by the Psychopathy Checklist List – Revised (PCL-R). This reliance is not without scrutiny, as researchers have noted several concerns. The assertion that the original factor structure of the checklist is viewed

---

Due to length limitations, all conceptualizations and their complementary measures of psychopathy are not covered. The measures covered herein represent widely researched, well-validated, and/or popular contemporary assessments of the construct of psychopathy. Beyond original scale revisions, their progeny measures will not be covered.

T. D. Kennedy et al., *Working with Psychopathy*, SpringerBriefs in Psychology,
https://doi.org/10.1007/978-3-030-84025-9_2

as commensurate with psychopathy, despite potentially inadequate coverage of all components of the construct (Skeem & Cooke, 2010), is one area of controversy among researchers. Other viable concerns revolve around the dimensionality of the construct (e.g., Guay et al., 2007) and the role of antisociality (e.g., Skeem & Cooke, 2010) and potentially adaptive traits (e.g., Patrick et al., 2013).

Contemporary theories, such as the triarchic model (Patrick et al., 2009) and psychopathy from the perspective of the five-factor model (FFM; McCrae & Costa, 1990) of personality (Widiger & Lynam, 1998), have sought to address limitations in the literature and practice. Although extant research is far from a unified conclusion in describing the construct of psychopathy, this chapter serves to provide an overview of psychopathic traits as defined by various psychopathy conceptualizations and their complementary measures. While Hare's PCL-R remains the gold standard in forensic psychopathy assessment, other psychopathy models and instruments, such as the Levenson Self-Report of Psychopathy Scale (LSRP; Levenson et al., 1995), Psychopathic Personality Inventory (PPI; Lilienfeld & Andrews, 1996), TriPM (Patrick, 2010), and Elemental Psychopathy Assessment (EPA; Lynam et al., 2011), have demonstrated empirical support (Tables 2.1 and 2.2). Additionally, psychopathy within the context of the Dark Triad will be briefly discussed.

Table 2.1 Timeline of psychopathy measures

PCL	PCL-R	LSRP	PPI	PPI-R	TriPM	EPA
1980	1991	1995	1996	2005	2010	2011

Table 2.2 Comparison of factor structures of psychopathy measures

	Two factor	Three factor	Four factor
PCL-R	Interpersonal-affective (Factor 1) Antisocial lifestyle (Factor 2)	Interpersonal Affective Behavior	Interpersonal Affective Lifestyle Antisocial
LSRP	Primary (interpersonal-affective) Secondary (antisocial lifestyle)	Egocentric (Factor 1) Antisocial (Factor 2) Callous (Factor 3)	
PPI-R	Self-centered impulsivity Fearless dominance	Self-centered impulsivity Fearless dominance Coldheartedness	
TriPM		Boldness Meanness Fearlessness	
EPA			Antagonism Disinhibition Emotional stability Narcissism

Note: Factor structures presented include those most frequently presented in research

2.1   Psychopathy Checklist – Revised: PCL-R

2.1.1   Overview

The PCL-R (Hare 1991, 2003) is used in forensic, research, and clinical settings, and, in some jurisdictions, the measure is considered a component of "best practices" protocols (e.g., Khiroya et al., 2009). It is widely considered to be the gold standard for the assessment of psychopathy. The PCL-R became known as such following decades of empirical literature supporting its use and validation, particularly applied to criminal justice contexts. Compared to other measures of psychopathy, few scales have survived the rigorous psychometric analysis that the PCL-R has been subjected to, and thus clinical and forensic use of the measure has proliferated.

The original 22-item scale was developed by Hare (1980, 1985) for measuring the construct of psychopathy in criminal populations. This original PCL was then revised into a 20-item scale: the PCL-R (1991, 2003). Each item is scored on a 3-point scale (0, 1, or 2; definitely not present to definitely present), and a total PCL-R score is obtained by summing the scores for each item; four subscale (or facet) scores are also produced. Importantly, the total score represents a measure of the construct of psychopathy in the individual and does not provide an assessment of risk level. There is no cutoff score where psychopathy is reached, though researchers have found a score of 30 (out of 40) to be a useful threshold. Hare (2021) acknowledges this cutoff as a methodological accommodation meant to aid communication between researchers and cites this in his manuals (1991, 2003). Hare describes his conceptualization of psychopathy as:

> a clinical construct that includes a cluster of interpersonal, affective, lifestyle, and antisocial traits and behaviors, including deception, manipulation, irresponsibility, impulsivity, stimulation-seeking, poor behavioral controls, shallow affect, a lack of empathy, guilt, or remorse, and a range of unethical and antisocial behaviors, not necessarily criminal (Hare, 2021, p.63).

Typically, a semi-structured interview is conducted and combined with the review of file and collateral information for the evaluator to rate the individual on the traits and behaviors described by Hare, which are captured in the scale items. The features are organized under four major domains of interpersonal, affective, lifestyle, and antisocial features. Hare (2003) notes that if an interview is not possible, the PCL-R can be scored using only file and collateral information; however, this limits the evaluator's ability to gain a comprehensive picture of the individual's affective and interpersonal "style."

While the PCL-R was not designed to be a risk assessment tool, researchers and clinicians have observed a relationship between psychopathic traits and violence, such that psychopathy has been considered a risk factor for future violence across many populations (e.g., Dolan & Doyle, 2000; Forth, et al., 1990; Quinsey et al., 1995; Salekin et al., 1996). Evaluating the presence of psychopathic traits has served to aid in risk management and informing treatment.

2.1.2   Development and Original Validation

Inspired by Cleckley's (1941, 1976) seminal work in conceptualizing psychopathy, Hare, his colleagues, and his students sought out to develop a scale measuring the construct. Ultimately, the combination of Cleckley's work, Hare's empirical research and experience, and the research of other professionals led to the development of the PCL and the PCL-R. Their process included compiling a list of features associated with psychopathy, including attributes, behaviors, and indicants, but also counterindicants. In a reductive method, statistical analyses were conducted to reduce over 100 features into 22 features that were considered to most suitably distinguish the construct. Interestingly, while Cleckley asserted low anxiety to be a central aspect of psychopathy, none of the final 22 items that Hare arrived at measure the degree or absence of anxiety. In another departure from Cleckley's writings, which did not purport impulsivity as a fundamental feature of psychopathy, one of the 22 distinguishing features put forth by Hare in the PCL captured impulsivity.

In 1980, Hare published his first validation study using a sample of 143 white incarcerated males from prison in British Columbia in Canada. High inter-rater reliabilities and internal consistency alphas were reported, and the PCL was supported in the ability of its total scores to predict global ratings of psychopathy. A principal component analysis indicated a five-factor solution that has not dominated in research. Subsequent, larger studies examining psychometric properties of the PCL (Harpur et al., 1988; Harpur et al., 1989) supported a correlated, two-factor structure, consisting of interpersonal-affective (Factor 1) and antisocial lifestyle (Factor 2) domains in incarcerated males. The interpersonal-affective factor includes features such as manipulation, grandiosity, and "selfish, callous, and remorseless use of others," whereas the lifestyle/antisocial factor is comprised of impulsive, antisocial, parasitic, and externalizing traits that can be considered socially deviant in nature. The measure was also found to have uniformly high reliability, reported through inter-rater reliabilities and internal consistencies for both factors. Through these initial studies, the PCL was determined to be a homogeneous measure, capturing the unidimensional construct of psychopathy through two related, yet distinct, factors.

2.1.3   Revision and Subsequent Validations

Hare's (1980) PCL validation study revealed two of the 22 items (i.e., *previous diagnosis as psychopath (or similar), drug or alcohol abuse not direct cause of antisocial behavior*) to have comparatively low correlations with the total score and were subsequently removed from the measure. Additionally, a revision was made to an item concerning *irresponsible behavior as parent* and was expanded to capture irresponsible behavior in varied contexts. Other smaller clarifications to scoring and wording were made. The resulting 20-item measure was called the PCL-Revised (PCL-R; 1991, 2003).

2.1.3.1 Two- (But Also Four-) Factor Model

A 1990 (Hare et al.) study using a sample of 1281 male offenders and forensic psychiatric patients examined the psychometrics and factor structure of the revised measure. They asserted excellent psychometric properties (i.e., inter-rater reliability and internal consistency) and reported a similar correlated, two-factor solution as presented by Harpur et al. (1988), supporting interpersonal/affective and antisocial lifestyle factors.

The 2003 PCL-R manual reports reliability and validity based on a mixed-gender sample of 10,896 North American and European offenders and forensic patients. Internal consistency and inter-rater reliabilities were high. An expansion of the original two-factor structure is presented, such that the two factors become higher-order factors with four equally important lower-order factors (also known as facets): interpersonal, affective, lifestyle, and antisocial. The interpersonal facet, representing arrogant and deceitful disposition, along with the affective facet, representing a deficient affective experience, are subsumed under the interpersonal/affective factor (Factor 1). Accordingly, the lifestyle facet, representing parasitic, impulsive, and irresponsible behaviors, and the antisocial facet, representing criminal/socially deviant behavior, are subsumed under the lifestyle/antisocial factor (Factor 2). The two higher-order factors remain moderately correlated, and the four facets showed moderate correlation as well. Thus, psychopathy is depicted as the shared variability between four equally important facets.

Support for the four-factor structure has been asserted in multiple additional studies (e.g., Babiak et al., 2010; Vitacco et al., 2005). Using a diverse collection of large samples that included male and female offenders, as well as male forensic psychiatric patients, Neumann et al. (2007) conducted exploratory and confirmatory factor analyses (EFA and CFA, respectively) and further provide support for the conceptualization of a superordinate factor of psychopathy represented by four correlated facets. In 2008, Hare and Neumann analyzed North American data sets and found indication for a different, yet harmonious, model with two higher-order factors, both of which consist of two lower-order factors; they contend that the lower-order facets parallel those of the four-factor model. A meta-analysis of over 13,000 male offenders across the globe (i.e., in North America, South America, England, Europe) and just over 1000 female offenders in North America by Neumann et al. (2015) concluded generally good statistical fit for the four-factor model across samples.

2.1.3.2 Three Factor Model

Some researchers have disagreed on the factor structure of the PCL-R and have published support for varying models, including a three-factor model. Cooke and Michie's (2001) three-factor model is notably different from previous PCL models given their exclusion of antisocial items from their analyses. In this utilization of only 13 out of the 20 items, psychopathy is interpreted from a perspective of pathological personality rather than antisocial behavior. The researchers argued that the two-factor model was not statistically convincing, and, based on their findings, a three-factor model may provide a more adequate model of psychopathy. Their analyses provide evidence for three factors, consisting of an arrogant, deceitful *interpersonal* style, deficient *affective* experiences, and an impulsive, irresponsible *behavior* style. Additional support for the three-factor model has been reported in other studies (e.g., Hall et al., 2004; Skeem et al., 2003). In opposition, Hare and colleagues have argued that the authors did not have conceptual or empirical basis for their removal of the antisocial items (e.g., Hare, 2021; Neumann et al., 2007), the presence of which has become a central debate in the conceptualization of psychopathy.

2.1.3.3 To Be (Antisocial) or Not to Be (Antisocial)?

There is a great degree of overlap between the three- and four-factor models. The key difference between the models is the association of antisocial behavior to psychopathy. In the three-factor model, antisocial behavior is a correlate, or even consequence, of psychopathy, whereas the four-factor model suggests that such behavior is characteristic of psychopathy. While many researchers (e.g., Cooke & Michie, 2001; Hare & Neumann, 2010; Skeem & Cooke, 2010) support the relationship between psychopathy and antisocial behavior, a growing body of evidence suggests that antisociality is not an *inherent* and *unavoidable* consequence of psychopathy, as conceptualizations such as the "successful psychopath" have surfaced (see Benning et al., 2018).

2.1.4 Limitations and Concerns

Despite a breadth of supporting literature, Hare's conceptualization of psychopathy has not existed without scrutiny. One prominent concern pertains to the emphasis placed on antisocial behavior and criminality (Cooke & Michie, 2001; Skeem & Cooke, 2010). Another criticism is regarding the generalizability (e.g., external validity) of Hare's findings beyond criminal and forensic populations. In a nuanced perspective using item response theory to examine psychopathy via cultural lens, Fanti et al. (2018) suggest that cultural variables may influence which PCL-R items, facets, or factors best distinguish the construct in a particular context. Additionally, the practical limitations of the PCL-R (e.g., requiring a trained rater, approximately 90–120 minutes for a thorough interview, and corroborating information) have become of importance to researchers. Over time, additional conceptualizations and measures of psychopathy have been developed, some of which aimed to address limitations within Hare's conceptualization.

2.2 Levenson Self-Report of Psychopathy: LSRP

2.2.1 Overview

The LSRP (also called the Levenson Primary and Secondary Psychopathy Scales or LPSP; Levenson et al., 1995) contains 26 self-report items constructed to measure psychopathy in nonoffender samples, while also measuring areas akin to those assessed in the PCL–R. Each item on the LSRP is rated on a 4-point Likert scale (1 – *disagree strongly,* 2 – *disagree somewhat,* 3 – *agree somewhat,* 4 – *agree strongly*), producing a total score as well as scores on two scales, labeled Primary and Secondary. Similar to other psychopathy instruments, such as the PCL/PCL-R, there is no designated cutoff score.

2.2.2 Development and Original Validation

2.2.2.1 Levenson et al.'s Two-Factor Model

The LSRP was created with the PCL-R factor structure in mind. More specifically, the primary scales were designed to parallel the PCL-R's first factor (affective/interpersonal), and the secondary scales were created to capture the second PCL-R factor (antisocial/lifestyle). The designation of the subscales was based on Karpman's (1948) psychodynamic approach to psychopathic personality, in which he contended that psychopathy can be split into two etiologically distinct groups: primary or idiopathic psychopathy and secondary, or symptomatic, psychopathy. Primary psychopathy reflects the traditional understanding of the psychopath as a person *predisposed* to callousness and selfish manipulation of others, whereas secondary psychopathy reflects a "neurotic" and impulsive presentation in which the person acts deviantly due to *environmental* factors (Karpman, 1948). Although the two PCL-R factors have been found to be moderately correlated, Levenson et al. (1995), quite notably and against conceptual expectations, paralleled Karpman's (1948) *distinct* pathways of psychopathy to Hare's (1991, 2003) correlated (i.e., *not distinct*) factors.

Levenson et al.'s (1995) original validation study used a sample of 487 undergraduate students and reported a two-factor solution, with good internal consistency of the primary scale but less-than-adequate internal consistency of the Secondary scale. The scales were moderately correlated with each other, and as expected, the Primary scale was observed to only slightly (positively) relate to trait anxiety, whereas the Secondary scale significantly positively related. While the modest correlation between scales conceptually aligns with the PCL-R-based construction of the LSRP, issue is drawn with Levenson et al.'s comparison of Primary and Secondary scales to Karpman's (1948) etiological assertions. Additionally, while both scales were (positively) correlated with antisocial actions, the Primary psychopathy scale reflected a stronger association with antisocial actions than the Secondary scale did, contrary to expectations. With the caveat that only persons with a high level of psychopathic features would qualify as psychopaths in forensic settings, based on their ability to identify a normal distribution of psychopathic traits (in both scales) in a noninstitutionalized population, the researchers contend that the construct of psychopathy is a continuous dimension and the LSRP shows promise as a self-report measure of psychopathy in said populations.

Recently, Sellbom et al. (2018) provided a comparison of effect sizes from multiple studies reporting associations between the Primary scale and extra-test psychopathy criteria, where they highlighted that said scale has reflected stronger associations with *behavioral* characteristics compared to associations with *affective-interpersonal* traits, which is contradictory to the intended construction of the Primary scale as corresponding to Hare's (1991, 2003) Factor 1 (interpersonal/ affective). From this standpoint, the construct validity of the LSRP has been called into question across multiple empirical examinations.

2.2.2.2   Lynam et al.'s Modified Two-Factor Model

Similar alphas to Levenson et al. (1995) were reported in a larger study of 1958 undergraduate participants (Lynam et al., 1999), which also supported the two-factor structure, this time through confirmatory factor analysis. In said factor analysis, a few modifications were made (e.g., correlating 17 residual errors and allowing Item 26 to load onto both factors, based on their analysis) that improved a poor model fit to an excellent one. The researchers noted that for each correlated residual error, it was clear that content beyond that which related to psychopathy was being shared. Like Levenson et al., the two LSRP scales were moderately correlated. This modest correlation reported between the two LSRP scales speaks to convergent validity *if* the two scales are considered lower-order factors of a psychopathy construct. However, concerns over discriminant validity arise when the two scales are viewed through the distinct etiological perspective asserted by Levenson et al. (1995). Lynam and colleagues' argued evidence of such discriminant validity through a pattern of correlational results between the two LSRP scales and the Big Five Inventory (BFI; John et al., 1991). In their examination of construct validity, all three LSRP scores were significantly correlated with lifetime and past-year serious delinquency and drug use, alcohol use in the past year, and history of arrest. Overall, Lynam et al. contend that the LSRP can be reliably and validly used to measure psychopathy in noninstitutionalized individuals.

2.2.2.3   From a Two-Factor Model to Maybe a Three-Factor Model? (Déjà Vu, Anyone?)

Contradicting previous interpretations of the LSRP's factor structure, a three-factor model (using only 19 of 26 original items) was first proposed through an exploratory factor analysis by Brinkley et al. (2008) using 430 federally incarcerated females. A three-factor model was later supported by Sellbom (2011) using confirmatory factor analysis with a sample of just over 400 male and female college students and nearly 600 male correctional inmates.

In Brinkley et al. (2008), the three identified factors were considered: Egocentric, Antisocial, and Callous, or Factors 1, 2, and 3, respectively. Through this structure, the Primary interpersonal/affective factor from prior studies appeared to have split into Egocentric and Callous factors, though analyses did not suggest that the two scales measured *precisely* the same construct identified in Levenson et al.'s (1995) Primary scale. However, the Antisocial factor was found to correspond well to Levenson et al.'s (1995) Secondary factor. Brinkley et al. reported internal consistencies for each scale, with only the Egocentric scale showing a strong Cronbach's alpha while the remaining two scales reflected alphas modestly below industry standard for adequacy. Concurrent validity was supported most strongly by the Antisocial scale, evidenced by higher scores on said scale to be associated with associations with a host of aversive psychological and legal outcomes. Overall, Brinkley et al. (2008) concluded the LSRP, while imperfect, is a reliable and valid self-report measure that may reflect a three-factor structure in, at least, incarcerated female populations.

Sellbom (2011) provided evidence supporting construct validity for the LSRP total and three-factor scores by demonstrating a promising pattern of convergent and discriminant validity (albeit with a few prominent exceptions). Convergent validity of the truncated 19-item measure did not suffer by removal of the same seven items from Brinkley et al. (2008). Sellbom (2011) could not, however, provide evidence of discriminant validity for the Antisocial factor scores, as the factor displayed moderate to large correlations with emotional distress, although the Egocentricity and Callous factor scores generally related to said criteria as expected (e.g., weakly). All three factors otherwise were interpreted to show a hopeful pattern of differential associations with conceptually relevant extra-test variables. Of concern, Sellbom (2011) reported weak correlations between the LSRP total score to measures of fearlessness and callousness/low empathy, though the total score was otherwise strongly related to all other conceptually expected measures evaluated. Internal consistencies measured by Cronbach's alpha for each score reflected a similar pattern to relevant previous studies. Nevertheless, Sellbom (2011) asserts promising evidence of the LSRP to measure psychopathy through a three-factor structure.

Across several follow-up studies, internal consistencies for the subscales have generally reflected the strongest values for Egocentricity, followed fairly closely by the Antisociality and Callousness scales (Anderson et al., 2013; Brinkley et al., 2008; Few et al., 2013; Sellbom, 2011; Sellbom & Phillips, 2013). Other studies have also found support for a three-factor model to the LSRP, using large community samples in the United States (Christian & Sellbom, 2016) and Italy (Somma et al., 2014) and large university samples in China (Shou et al., 2016) and the United States (Salekin et al., 2014). Investigations into concurrently validity have found a significant association with the LSRP and PCL-R, though the LSRP has generally reflected smaller correlations to the PCL-R when compared to other self-report psychopathy measures (e.g., the PPI in Berardino et al., 2005; the LSRP in Lilienfeld & Andrews, 1996).

2.2.3   Limitations, Concerns, and an Expanded Measure?

Given the discrepancies in literature concerning the best fitting model of the LSRP, clear and confident claims regarding the factor structure of the LSRP cannot be asserted. Studies have provided evidence questioning the construct validity of the Primary scale, given stronger associations observed with antisocial behaviors than interpersonal and affective traits (e.g., Lilienfeld & Hess, 2001; Poythress et al. 2010). Additionally, results that question the ability of the Primary scale to capture characteristics such as fearlessness and low empathy (Sellbom, 2011) are of exceptional concern to Levenson et al.' (1995) original intent for the scale to assess primary features of psychopathy as portrayed by Karpman (1948). While the LSRP provides hope toward the self-reported measurement of psychopathy, some room was left for improvement.

In 2016, Christian and Sellbom introduced an expanded version of the LSRP that was partially intended to address some of the previously noted psychometric issues, particularly regarding construct validity. Ten items were added to improve construct coverage, resulting in a 36-item measure. The original 4-point Likert scale was expanded to a 6-point scale (1 *strongly disagree*, 2 *disagree*, 3 *somewhat disagree*, 4 *somewhat agree*, 5 *agree*, 6 *strongly agree*). Their validation study consisted of large sample of community participants and, in comparison to the original LSRP, reported stronger evidence of convergent and discriminant validity. The expanded scale also exhibited better internal consistency and construct validity than the original LSRP.

To date, only one additional study (Maheux-Caron et al., 2020) has examined this expanded version of the LSRP (Christian & Sellbom, 2016), though the study was conducted with a French adaptation of said scale on 432 French Canadian community participants. The measure was found to have generally comparable psychometric properties to the original expanded LSRP and was interpreted as an appropriate option in research and screening contexts within French-speaking communities.

2.3   Psychopathic Personality Inventory – Revised: PPI-R

2.3.1   Overview

The PPI-R is one of the most extensively studied self-report measures of psychopathy. Unlike the PCL-R, the PPI-R was created for use with noncriminal populations, though studies have also supported its use with forensic (i.e., criminal and psychiatric) populations (Poythress et al., 1998; Poythress et al., 2010). The scale purports to measure psychopathic personality traits through a dimensional, rather than a taxonic, perspective. The original 187-item scale was published by Lilienfeld and Andrews in 1996 and was revised in 2005 into a 154-item scale: the PPI-R (Lilienfeld & Widows). Each item is scored on a 4-point scale (*false*, *mostly false*, *mostly true*, or *true*), and a total score is obtained by summing the scores for each item. Eight subscale scores are also calculated, in the areas of Machievellian Egocentricity (30 items), Social Potency (24 items; later renamed *Social Influence* in PPI-R), Coldheartedness (21 items), Carefree Nonplanfulness (20 items), Fearlessness (19 items), Blame Externalization (18 items), Impulsive Nonconformity (17 items), and Stress Immunity (11 items). Finally, three-factor scores are also calculated in the domains of Self-Centered Impulsivity, Fearless Dominance, and Coldheartedness.

2.3.2   Development and Original Validation

Lilienfeld and Andrews (1996) developed the PPI following various concerns and gaps in the conceptualization of psychopathy. Unsurprisingly, the researchers cited trepidation with the applicability of the PCL-R outside of criminal populations. They considered the importance of understanding a subclinical expression of psychopathy, which they argued would not have been captured in research with incarcerated populations. Additionally, the PCL-R being a time-consuming measure scored through interview and file review encouraged Lilienfeld and Andrews (1996) to produce a tool that was befitting for large-scale research beyond prison walls.

Using an exploratory approach and driven by theory and literature, Lilienfeld and Andrews (1996) produced a pool of items that was related to psychopathy. Notably, in contrast to other self-report measures of psychopathy that specify the assessment of antisocial behaviors, Lilienfeld and Andrews focused on personality constructs and intentionally avoided reliance on capturing explicit antisocial behavior. The wording of their items was crafted to minimize social undesirability and to seem generally normative, given that their intent was to measure psychopathy within community populations. Through iterative and self-correcting exploratory methods, the researchers arrived at the aforementioned eight content scales that comprise the PPI.

Lilienfeld and Andrews (1996) used five undergraduate samples to first examine the psychometric properties of their measure. Making a similar conceptual leap to Levenson et al. (1995) regarding dimensionality, the assumption of psychopathy as being dimensional (versus taxonic) was made and explicitly announced by the researchers (explained by their use of undergraduate samples). The PPI total score and its eight subscales reflected acceptable to high reliability, as measured by internal consistency and test-rest reliability. Additionally, Lilienfeld and Andrews (1996) report on four studies that found evidence of convergent and discriminant validity in the measure and its subscales, across different rating methods (i.e., self-report, interview, observational, and archival). Support for incremental validity relative to other utilized self-report psychopathy-associated measures (e.g., the MMPI Psychopathic Deviate and MMPI-2 Antisocial Practices content scales) was also reported. In terms of construct validity, the researchers indicated promising, albeit preliminary, findings regarding its assessment with noncriminal populations.

Of conceptual concern, however, was the identification of low negative correlations between many PPI subscales, notably those measuring features of negative affectivity (primarily, Blame Externalization and Stress Immunity scales) (Lilienfeld & Andrews, 1996). An implication of this could be that psychopathy is not a "classical syndrome" in which a similar constellation of signs and symptoms is found across psychopaths (Lilienfeld, 2013). Along with identifying preliminary support for the PPI, Lilienfeld and Andrews cautioned readers in viewing *any* psychopathy measure, including theirs, as a complete delineation of all relevant psychopathic traits, given their conceptualization that the construct of psychopathy holds an indeterminate number of indictors.

The factor structure of the PPI was examined by Benning et al. (2003) using a community sample of 353 individual male twins. Their findings presented an uncorrelated two-factor solution consisting of Fearless Dominance (Stress Immunity, Fearlessness, and Social Potency scales) and Impulsive Antisociality (Blame Externalization, Machiavellian Egocentricity, Impulsive Nonconformity, and Carefree Nonplanfulness scales), later called Self-Centered Impulsivity. Confidence in their factor structure interpretation is made questionable when one considers the substantial cross-loading of the Fearlessness subscale, and lesser-yet-notable cross-loading of the Stress Immunity scale, onto the second factor, when they conceptually "belong" to the first factor; similar problematic cross-loadings were observed by Benning et al. (2005). Additionally, the Coldheartedness content scale was not found to load substantially on either factor, and some literature has thus considered Coldheartedness to be a distinct domain measured by the PPI (Benning et al., 2005; Berg et al., 2015). Ultimately, the current conceptualization of the scale remains unclear, and additional clarifying studies are warranted.

While studies using nonoffender (e.g., Benning et al., 2005; Witt et al., 2009a, b), offender (e.g., Edens & McDermott, 2010), and combined samples (Ross et al., 2009) have replicated the two-factor structure reported by Benning et al. (2003), as commonplace in scientific research, conflicting literature has been published. Using data drawn from 1224 male inmates, Neumann et al. (2008) were unable to replicate the original two-factor model. In its place, they proposed a three-factor structure with the content scales loading as follows: Fearlessness, Impulsive Noncomformity, Machiavellian Egocentricity, and Blame Externalization loaded on the first factor, Stress Immunity and Social Potency loaded onto the second factor, and the remaining scales, Carefree Nonplanfulness, and Coldheartedness loaded onto the third factor. The factors were not named. In conclusion, the researchers do not deter others from using the PPI despite the current study's inability to support Benning et al.'s (2003) two-factor structure in an offender sample and further indicate that the PPI maintains promise in conceptualizing psychopathy—though, by way of how many dimensions are unclear.

Recently, Ruchensky et al. (2018) offered a possible account for the divergent findings regarding factor structures of the PPI (and PPI-R): sample type. Noting that the validation studies (in support of two higher order factors) used noncriminal samples whereas studies supporting a three-factor solution (Lilienfeld &Widows, 2005; Neumann et al., 2008) used criminal samples, the researchers examined the role of sample type as a moderator of the measure's factor structure. After performing a meta-analytic factor analysis using over 18,000 participants, Ruchensky et al. (2018) reported evidence that the properties (i.e., the factor structure) of the PPI/PPI-R vary based on whether individuals are from an offending or community population. More specifically, a two-factor model (similar to Benning et al., 2003) consisting of Self-Centered Impulsivity and Fearless Dominance was generally supported in community samples. Offender samples, instead, better fit a three-factor model of Self-Centered Impulsivity, Fearless Dominance, and Coldheartedness; however, the Fearlessness subscale, interestingly, loaded on the Self-Centered Impulsivity Factor (and not Fearless Dominance). In the offender sample, the Stress Immunity scale was more negatively correlated (compared to nonoffenders) with externalizing measures, indicating that resistance to stress is protective against externalizing behaviors in offenders. The authors explained that the differences between populations were highlighted in arguably adaptive traits, such as the minimal need for a recovery period in the context of a stressful situation.

2.3.3   Revision and Subsequent Validations

In 2005, the PPI was revised (Lilienfeld & Widows) by means of removal of certain items (i.e., cultural-specific items and items with problematic psychometrics) and a reduction in the reading level required for the measure. Newly introduced to the PPI-R were four validity scales: two measured Inconsistent Responding and the other two assessed for Deviant Responding and Virtuous Responding. The final 154-item measure, scored on the original 4-point Likert scale, was named the PPI-R and is otherwise structurally similar to the original scale. The PPI-R contains the familiar eight subscales (i.e., Blame Externalization, Machiavellian Egocentricity, Impulsive Nonconformity, Carefree Nonplanfulness, Stress Immunity, Fearlessness, Social Influence (renamed from Social Potency), and Coldheartedness) that load onto three higher-order factors (i.e., Self-Centered Impulsivity, Fearless Dominance, and Coldheartedness). Scoring results in one total, three factor, and eight subscale scores (note: the Coldheartedness factor score is also the Coldheartedness subscale score).

Lilienfeld and Widows (2005) examined two samples, community/college and offender, in their validation study. Internal consistency coefficients for total and subscale scores supported reliability of the scores in both samples (the mean alpha coefficients for the factor scores were slightly higher for the community/college sample). Test-retest reliability was also assessed for total, subscale, and factor scores and reflected strong reliability values.

Other studies have reported similar and sometimes better reliability properties (e.g., Anestis et al., 2011; Seibert et al., 2011) of the PPI-R. An exploration into the measure's construct validity using forensic psychiatric participants (Edens & McDermott, 2010) discovered a relationship between Self-Centered Impulsivity factor scores and antisocial outcomes (e.g., substance abuse, risk for violence, hostility and anger, overall psychiatric symptoms). In contrast, alcohol abuse/dependence, depression, low anxiety, and anger were predicted by the Fearless Dominance factor. Regarding convergent and discriminant validity, evidence of such in the PPI-R has been reported in analyses using the LSRP (Lilienfeld & Widows, 2005).

2.3.4 The Fearless Dominance Debate

The matter of adaptive traits (e.g., stress immunity, social poise, and emotional resilience) and their place in the nomological network of psychology remains unresolved within the literature. These adaptive traits, captured within the Fearless Dominance domain of the PPI/PPI-R, have also been described using the term "boldness" (see Patrick et al., 2009). The debate was ignited, in part, by Miller and Lynam (2012) observations of weak relationships between social and physical boldness (as measured through the Fearless Dominance subscale of the PPI-R) and PCL-R scores (total and factor); similar findings were reported by Marcus et al. (2013). A potential explanation exists, however, that the PCL-R was developed on criminal populations, and thus less attention may have been afforded to capturing adaptive traits in the measure. Miller and Lynam further emphasize the scientific debate by finding weak associations between the Fearless Dominance domain and measures of externalizing and antisocial behaviors.

While disagreement for the role of Fearless Dominance has been presented in these and other studies (e.g., Crego & Widiger, 2014), researchers such as Lilienfeld et al. (2016), Patrick et al. (2013), and Berg et al. (2017) have explicitly voiced support for the central role of boldness traits in the conceptualization of psychopathy. Lilienfeld et al. provided evidence for their endorsement through a meta-analytic examination of adaptive traits as measured domains within the PPI and TriPM, in comparison to non-PCL-R measures of psychopathy (e.g., EPA; Youth Psychopathic Traits Inventory: Andershed et al., 2002). By using non-PCL-R measures, Lilienfeld et al. attempted to address the potential issue surrounding the PCL-R's validation with criminal populations and decreased emphasis on adaptive features relevant to psychopathy.

2.3.5 Limitations and Concerns

While Ruchensky et al.'s (2018) recent meta-analysis suggests that the most appropriate factor structure of the PPI/PPI-R is moderated by sample type, questions remain. For example, the researchers offer that the moderating effect of sample could potentially point to genuine, personality differences, but it could otherwise suggest a response driven by situational factors (such as within the legal system). Implications for research, intervention, and assessment are significant if the conceptualization of psychopathy can elucidate whether such observed differences are personality or situationally based. Further, pivotal questions surround the role of adaptive features, such as those represented by the Fearless Dominance domain. Beyond conceptualization matters, the PPI-R is a self-report measure and is thus not immune to the commonly noted concerns with this method of data collection (e.g., the inherent challenge in insightfully and genuinely measurement traits representing psychopathy due to factors such as manipulation and/or lack of insight; see Lilienfeld & Fowler, 2006).

2.4 Triarchic Psychopathy Measure: TriPM

2.4.1 Overview

The Triarchic Psychopathy Measure (Patrick, 2010) was developed based on the triarchic model put forth by Patrick et al. (2009). The TriPM is a 58-item self-report measure comprised of three scales (i.e., Boldness, Meanness, Disinhibition). The Boldness scale contains 19 items, whereas the Meanness and Disinhibition scales contain 19 and 20 items, respectively. Each item is rated on a 4-point Likert scale (*true, somewhat true, somewhat false, false*). Three domain scores are produced, with no cutoff points or descriptors of the domain scores; higher scores are simply explained to be more indicative of psychopathic features. The measure was developed specifically for research purposes and is not meant to be a diagnostic and/or risk assessment tool.

2.4.2   Development and Original Validation

Inspired by research findings that boldness explains a key difference between psychopathy and antisocial personality disorder (Wall et al., 2015), the developers of the triarchic model argue that Hare's measure does not (fully) capture all elements of psychopathy, particularly boldness. Like other researchers, they, too, were concerned about the PCL-R's focus on criminality. Further, Patrick et al. (2012) assert that PCL-R does not measure distinct constructs. In light of the noted empirical issues, and with the intent to integrate empirically germane domains, Patrick et al. (2009) proposed the triarchic model which asserts three core constructs of psychopathy: Boldness (the integration of high dominance with low anxiousness and adventuresomeness), Meanness (characterized by an inclination for callousness, cruelty, and predatory aggression), and Disinhibition (the tendency for impulsiveness, irresponsibility, oppositionality, and angry/hostile behavior), which they proclaim to be intersecting, but distinct, phenotypic constructs. Rather than a heavy focus on criminality as they argue exists in the PCL-R, Patrick et al. (2009) placed an equal focus on all three of their proposed core constructs.

To operationalize and empirically test their model, the TriPM was developed (Patrick, 2010). The measure is comprised of three scales which index the proposed three core constructs. The Boldness scale is based on the operationalization of Fearless Dominance from the PPI-R, whereas items for the Meanness and Disinhibition scales were drawn from the Externalizing Spectrum Inventory, which comprehensively assesses externalizing traits and behaviors (ESI; Krueger et al., 2007).

Reported in the TriPM manual, Patrick (2010) compared the measure to the PCL-R and various extant self-report measures of psychopathy, in non-offenders (college), substance abuse treatment, and offender samples. Weak to modest intercorrelations between the Triarchic scales were reported in prisoner and substance abuse treatment samples (totaling 326 male participants). However, this is expected given that Patrick (2010) indicates the scales are meant to represent three distinct constructs, but with intersecting components. Unfortunately, Patrick (2010) does not analyze any reliability coefficients. Reflecting concurrent validity, overall support for the measurement of psychopathic traits as compared to the PCL-R was reported using the same male offender sample, whereas support in comparison to the PPI was observed using a mixed-gender college sample of 631 participants (Patrick, 2010). While the absence of large correlations between the PCL-R and TriPM was observed, the interpretation is offered, such that this is to be expected given the different measurement contexts: the PCL-R is a clinical diagnostic tool, whereas the TriPM is scored on self-report only, and correlational strength can be negatively impacted when measuring the same construct under divergent methods (Campbell & Fiske, 1959). In contrast, all Triarchic scales displayed moderate to large associations with most of the self-report measures (i.e., the PPI, the SRP-III; Paulhus et al., 2016, and the YPI; Andershed et al., 2002), although not the LSRP.

Examination of PCL-R and TriPM regression betas reflected an association between each TriPM scale and a lower-order facet from the PCL-R (Patrick, 2010). More specifically, the Boldness, Meanness, and Disinhibition scales were reported to be most related to the PCL-R's Interpersonal, Affective, and Lifestyle facets, respectively. Patrick (2010) noted that the three scales individually contribute to the prediction of the PCL-R Antisocial Behavior facet, implying that boldness, meanness, and disinhibition tendencies assert a combinative influence in maintaining criminal behavior. Together, the Triarchic scales predict overall PCL-R scores to a high degree, despite individual scales showing only modest correlations with total PCL-R scores.

2.4.3 Subsequent Validations

Researchers have found good to excellent inter-rater reliabilities and test-retest reliabilities (Sellbom & Phillips, 2013; Stanley et al., 2013; Blagov et al., 2016) of TriPM scores. Stanley et al. (2013) also found support for construct validity using an offender sample of 141 participants. Based on data from incarcerated females and undergraduate students, Sellbom and Phillips (2013) found that the triarchic scales demonstrated conceptually consistent relationships to other measures of psychopathy (i.e., PPI-R, LSRP, APSD – Youth version; Frick & Hare, 2001) further supporting construct validity.

Research on the factor structure of the TriPM reflects mixed findings. Drislane and Patrick (2017) found support for a three-factor model fit based on CFA results. Using data from over 1000 Italian-dwelling community adults, Somma et al. (2019) also supported a three-factor structure through CFA and exploratory structural equation model (ESEM) analyses. Item-level structural examination of the TriPM was interpreted to be in general alignment with the domains of boldness, meanness, and disinhibition. A similar three-factor interpretation was offered by Latzman et al. (2019) using ESEM analysis on data from nearly 500 undergraduate and community participants.

Nevertheless, some studies have reported results that draw concern with the three-factor model. For instance, Shou et al. (2018), using a Chinese sample and a Chinese version of the TriPM, assert that the three domains are comprised of subdimensions. Additionally, despite Somma et al.'s (2019) support for a three-factor model, problems related to certain item loadings were identified (i.e., a Meanness item loaded onto the Boldness and Disinhibition factors), and the researchers had to account for potentially meaningful variance that was not drawn from the three factors.

2.4.4 Alternative Factor Structures

Roy et al. (2021) and Collison et al. (2021) identified more than three factors in their structural analyses of the TriPM. Using over 1000 community participants, Roy et al. found evidence for seven factors through EFA and CFA analyses, thus reframing the Triarchic model to a septarchic one. Most of the Boldness scale items loaded onto Positive Self-image, Leadership, and Stress Immunity factors, whereas most of the Meanness and Disinhibition items loaded onto the Callousness and Enjoy Hurting and trait Impulsivity and overt Antisociality factors, respectively. Further, Roy et al. report evidence of multidimensionality within each triarchic scale. They conclude that the three-factor model is not a statistically appropriate representation of the triarchic model. Collison et al. (2021) analyzed data from 431 adults and instead asserted support for a six-factor model comprised of: Antisociality, Stress Immunity, Callousness, Leadership, Sensation Seeking, and Impulsivity factors. Again, Collison et al.'s findings were not without concerns of multidimentionality and problematic loadings.

Most recently, Stanton et al. (2021) and Eichenbaum et al. (2021) conducted item-level factor structure analyses of the TriPM. Stanton et al. analyzed community and undergraduate samples (over 1200 participants) and were able to replicate a three-factor model through EFA but not CFA. Similar to other studies (e.g., Latzman et al., 2019, Somma et al., 2019), many items reflected problematic loadings, particularly in the Meanness scale. Guided by their factor analytic results, the researchers removed items (going from 58 to 35) across all scales that were not clear indicators of its assigned domain and used alternate scoring for the three scales. The alternate domain scores were interpreted to better represent the traditional triarchic dimensions as the alternate scores. Through this analytic lens, they conclude that their briefer "Alternate TriPM" may be viable avenue of assessing triarchic domains.

Eichenbaum et al. (2021) conducted EFAs on data from 937 college and community members and found unidimensional support for the Disinhibition and Meannness scales but asserted evidence of dimensionality in the Boldness scale, best characterized by two domains. All three scales were observed to have items that had minimal ability to discriminate between participants who held varying levels of the trait in question. Of concern, differential item functioning between sexes was observed in 61% of the items, spanning across all scales, meaning that men and women who held similar levels of the trait were found to have responded differently to the same items. The authors conclude that the TriPM performed better at measuring disinhibition and meanness in persons with high levels of the traits than it did persons with lower levels of the boldness trait, with the caveat that the TriPM fails to measure said traits equally between sexes.

2.4.5 Limitations and Concerns

Being a self-report measure without validity scales, the TriPM is not immune to the limitations commonly ascribed to self-report measures of psychopathy (e.g., impression management, feigning, lack of insight to facilitate accurate responding). Of greater concern, evidence of multidimensionality within triarchic scales, troubling psychometrics properties, and debates over the underlying factor structure of the TriPM currently characterize the state of research on the TriPM. Although Patrick (2010) explained that the Boldness domain alone cannot capture psychopathy and it must be considered with the other two TriPM domains, a central debate in psychopathy literature concerns the extent to which the adaptive trait of Boldness (or Fearless Dominance, as measured by the PPI) is (or is not) a central component of psychopathy (e.g., Crowe et al., 2021; Miller & Lynam, 2012). While the TriPM continues to gain interest, the measure requires additional empirical support and structural clarification before it can become the next widely recognized and validated self-report measure of psychopathy.

2.5 Elemental Psychopathy Assessment: EPA

2.5.1 Overview

Another attempt at reconciling questions with Hare's and other scholars' conceptualizations of psychopathy has been made with the consideration of psychopathy within the five-factor model of personality (Lynam & Widiger, 2007; Miller et al., 2001; Widiger & Lynam, 1998), measured through the Elemental Psychopathy Assessment (Lynam et al., 2011). Widiger and Lynam contend that because of its limitations, the PCL-R's factor structure may not reveal all foundational elements of psychopathy. The researchers further question the belief that psychopathy is a homogenous condition and argue that it can be embedded and studied within the framework of a validated and comprehensive model of personality, particularly, the five-factor model (FFM: McCrae & Costa, 1990). The FFM posits that personality can be defined through five major domains of Openness to Experience, Conscientiousness, Extraversion, Agreeableness, and Neuroticism. Widiger and Lynam argue that psychopathy is an "extreme variant of a common, fundamental dimension of personality" (pp. 182) and thus conceptualize it through this lens. Rather than posing psychopathy as a homogenous, pathological departure from typical personality functioning, it is considered a heterogenous constellation of normal personality traits. More specifically, the defining aspects of psychopathy include low Agreeableness and low Conscientiousness, though psychopathic traits are also drawn from the other FFM dimensions. Further empirical evidence in support of the perspective that psychopathy can be measured through the FFM has since been published (e.g., Lynam & Widiger, 2007; Miller et al., 2001).

2.5.2 Development and Initial Validation

The FFM is not a scale like the TriPM or PCL-R, and unlike the triarchic model, the FFM purports to explain personality as a whole. The EPA, however, is based on the FFM, and its operationalized measure: the NEO Personality Inventory–Revised (NEO-PI–R; Costa & McCrae, 1992). This was developed by Lynam et al. (2011) to evaluate psychopathy through personality elements obtained through self-report. The EPA was constructed to have the capability of measuring "extreme" variants of normal personal traits, as Widiger and Lynam (1998) argued to exist in psychopathy. Using facets of the NEO PI-R that were previously indicated as characteristic of psychopathy (Lynam & Widiger, 2007), the EPA's authors wrote items that were meant to represent each facet, but with pathological or maladaptive descriptions (e.g., "My stubbornness has frequently gotten me into trouble") beyond what exists in the NEO PI-R. Explicit antisocial content, though, was excluded. The final measure included 178 items, and scoring produces two validity scale scores, a total score, four factor scores (Antagonism, Disinhibition, Emotional Stability, and Narcissism; Few et al., 2013), and 18 subscale (or facet) scores: Unconcern, Anger-Hostility, Self-Contentment, Self-Assurance, Urgency, Invulnerability, Coldness, Dominance, Thrill-Seeking, Distrust, Manipulation, Self-Centeredness, Opposition, Arrogance, Callousness, Disobliged, Impersistence, and Rashness (Lynam et al., 2011).

In the original validation using three undergraduate samples, Lynam et al. (2011) concluded the EPA's scales as unidimensional and internally consistent. Further, strong associations between the EPA scales and their original FFM counterpart scales were observed, and incremental validity over NEO PI-R scores of psychopathy was also reported; EPA scales, overall, out predicted the NEO PI–R scales in analyses with the SRP-III, LSRP, and PPI-R. The EPA's total score was also significantly associated with the same three measures. A joint factor analysis including both NEO PI-R and EPA facets revealed the anticipated five-factor structure of general personality and, in most cases, highest loadings of EPA scales onto their original FFM domains. The same researchers found strong convergent validity with SRP-III and EPA total scores using a sample of 70 male inmates. EPA total scores in this sample were also substantially correlated with disciplinary infractions, antisocial behavior, and alcohol use. Overall, initial psychometric examinations of the EPA reflected encouraging findings.

2.5.3 Subsequent Validations

Wilson et al. (2011) contributed psychometric information pertaining to the EPA's construct validity, also using undergraduate participants. Findings included a strong internal consistency alpha for the total score and generally satisfactory to strong alphas for the four-factor scales, though the Arrogance scale just failed to meet the desired threshold for acceptability. Substantial convergence between the EPA total scale scores and scores from other psychopathy measures (i.e., PPI-R, LSRP, and SRP-III) was found. Further evidence of construct validity was found by Miller et al. (2011a, b) using a mixed-gender sample of 227 undergraduates. Overall, EPA scores were observed to be correlated in expectant ways to psychopathy-related constructs (e.g., narcissism, antisocial behaviors), and most of the EPA facets (13 out of 18) showed strong associations with their derivative FFM domains. However, attention was drawn to the EPA total score's lack of association with the Neuroticism domain. Miller et al. argue that certain EPA scores were significantly related (positively and negatively) to Neuroticism, thus masking a significant level of heterogeneity in the relationship. The positive relationship was observed between EPA scales concerning externalizing behaviors and measures of anger and aggression, whereas EPA scales relating to resiliency toward negative emotions were conversely related to the same measures. Based on other studies' similar findings of commonly null correlations between arguably adaptive psychopathic traits (e.g., fearless dominance/boldness) and externalizing behaviors (Skeem & Cooke, 2010), future studies are encouraged to closely examine the lower-order facets of psychopathy.

Investigating the factor structure of the 18 subscales of the EPA, Few et al. (2013) used two university samples and identified four factors: Antagonism (Factor 1), Emotional Stability (Factor 2), Disinhibition (Factor 3), and Narcissism (Factor 4). The Antagonism and Emotional Stability factors were comprised of scales relating to the FFM domain of Agreeableness (reverse scored) and Neuroticism (reverse scored), respectively. The third factor, Disinhibition, was identified through scales regarding maladaptive variants of the FFM domain of Conscientiousness, whereas the fourth factor, Narcissism, was comprised of a variety of EPA scales corresponding to multiple FFM domains: Extraversion, Agreeableness, and Neuroticism, with the latter two reverse scored. In this way, the psychopathic personality is demonstrated through lower levels of agreeableness, neuroticism, and conscientiousness, and higher degrees of extraversion. Additionally, convergent validity was supported in examination of the SRP-III, PPI-R, and LSRP to the EPA total and factor scores, though in contexts of SRP-III and LSRP, little convergence was observed with the EPA Emotional Stability factor. One reason for this may be due to a lower emphasis placed on adaptive traits, given that the SRP-III (a PCL-R derivative) and LSRP were developed based on the PCL-R. Depending on one's perspective on the importance (or lack thereof) of adaptive features in conceptualizing psychopathy, the EPA might therefore be considered a more comprehensive assessment of psychopathy than measures which neglect the central role of said traits.

To build upon prior literature primarily sampling undergraduates, Miller et al. (2014) gathered data from 104 community members who were oversampled for psychopathic traits. They reported high alphas for all four factor scores and the total score. Construct and criterion validity was supported through the comparison of EPA scores with self- and informant-rated SRP-III scores, as well as with dimensions from the HEXACO model of personality, the Narcissistic Personality Inventory (NPI; Raskin & Terry, 1988), a measure of Machiavellianism – the MACH-IV (Christie & Geis, 1970), and externalizing behaviors (e.g., antisocial behavior, aggression). Moderate to strong correlations were consistently identified between the SPR-III scores and EPA factors; however, like Few et al. (2013), only limited convergence was reported between the Emotional Stability factor of the EPA and SRP-III scales. Further, none of the EPA factors showed significant interactions with the EPA Emotional Stability factor, again drawing empirical attention (e.g., Lilienfeld et al., 2012), to the question of adaptive traits in the conceptualization of psychopathy.

Concern in literature has been raised that persons with psychopathic traits (in non-forensic settings) are either unable or unwilling to accurately provide information regarding their psychopathic traits. Given the substantial convergence observed between self-report and informant reports of psychopathy in their findings, juxtaposed with findings from Miller et al. (2011a, b) and Ray et al. (2013), Miller and colleagues voice support for the use of self-report instruments in examining psychopathy, with a caveat: self-report instruments (across constructs) are inherently unsuitable for contexts in which the respondent has a significant incentive to respond deceivingly (e.g., custody cases). Miller et al. concluded that the EPA is a promising and comprehensive measure in the assessment of psychopathic traits.

2.5.4 Limitations and Concerns

The EPA is the newest addition to the self-report family of psychopathy scales and has thus far indicate generally good psychometric properties. Accordingly, while the research base is growing, it is limited. Existing studies reflect a promising future for the EPA, though researchers and evaluators should exercise caution until additional validation studies in support of the instrument accumulate. For instance, much more research is needed to further generalize the EPA's ability to measure psychopathy in populations other than community members and undergraduates, given only Lynam et al. (2011) has studied the EPA with a forensic population. Along the same lines, research in diverse populations and other countries is also called for. A specific need highlighted in the existing literature surrounds Emotional Stability scale and the role of adaptive traits in psychopathy. Finally, future factor analytic studies should also seek to replicate the EPA's four-factor structure via additional EFAs but also through CFA and using IRT.

2.5.4.1 Psychopathy Within (or Above?) the Dark Triad

Conceptualization of the Dark Triad intended to capture the malevolent side of human nature and includes constructs that have been empirically interpreted as unique but overlapping: Machiavellianism, subclinical narcissism, and subclinical psychopathy (Paulhus & Williams, 2002). Machiavellianism, or the manipulative personality, was proposed by Christie and Geis (1970) based on Machiavelli's statements (from his original books) that were distilled into normal personality items.

Machiavelli, a political advisor in the 1500s, is well known for his intimidating, violent, and amoral methods of achieving power. Within the Dark Triad, Machiavellianism is characterized as manipulative, cold, and lacking in conscientiousness (Paulhus & Williams). The MACH-IV, developed by Christie and Geis (1970), was originally used by Paulus and Williams to examine Machiavellianism as a construct within the Dark Triad.

Subclinical, or "normal," narcissism was proposed by Raskin and Hall (1979) through attempts to define a subclinical version of narcissistic personality disorder. Emphasis was placed on superiority, grandiosity, entitlement, and dominance facets of the clinical syndrome. Ultimately, the NPI was produced and had since been supported empirically (e.g., Kubarych et al., 2004; Raskin & Terry, 1988), though problematic research findings, such as controversies over factor structure, can easily be found (e.g., Ackerman et al., 2011; Brown et al., 2009). Paulhus and Williams (2002) used the NPI to capture narcissism within the Dark Triad.

Subclinical psychopathy within the triad includes central features such as high impulsivity and thrill-seeking, juxtaposed with low anxiety and empathy (Paulhus & Williams, 2002). Hare's SRP-III (a self-report of psychopathy) was used for the measurement of psychopathy within the Dark Triad, with the empirical defense that the measure has been validated in nonclinical samples (Forth et al., 1996). Together, the Dark Triad constructs of Machiavellianism, narcissism and psychopathy are originally measured across three distinct scales and totaling over 90 items.

To facilitate a more efficient measurement of Dark Triad constructs, two (separate) measures were developed: The Dirty Dozen (DD; Jonason & Webster, 2010) and the Short Dark Triad (SD3; Jones & Paulhus, 2014), consisting of 12 and 27 items, respectively. While validation efforts have revealed generally promising findings, the DD has been found to perform less optimally than the SD3 in terms of correlations with counterpart scales of MACH-IV, NPI, and SRP-III (Maples et al., 2014). While it was the basis for the construction of the scales, the limited set of items is, nevertheless, noted as a concern in both measures (e.g., Miller et al., 2012).

In Muris et al.'s (2017) meta-analysis of Dark Triad literature, they concluded that Dark Triad traits are significantly correlated, contradicting Paulhus and William's (2002) assertion that the constructs, while overlapping, are distinct. Differences between men and women on psychopathy only were identified (i.e., dark triad traits were more prevalent in men), and such traits are generally associated with diverse and negative psychosocial outcomes (e.g., interpersonal difficulties, aggression/delinquency, socioemotional deficits) (Muris et al.). These negative outcomes were found to correlate most convincingly with psychopathy over Machiavellianism and narcissism. Muris et al. question the inclusion of all three constructs and contend that psychopathy is the dominant trait in which to explain malevolent behavior. This contention is supported not only by their meta-analytic results but also in other studies reflecting psychopathy to be a unique predictor of various transgressions (e.g., financial misbehavior in Jones, 2014; cyberbullying in Goodboy & Martin, 2015; racism in Jonason, 2015).

Conceptualization of the Dark Triad of personality is an attractive and parsimonious effort at elucidating wicked and unscrupulous personalities. Be that as it may, the theoretical and empirical evidence behind the conceptualization is mixed, given the assertion that Machiavellianism and narcissism can be contained within psychopathy as a construct (e.g., Glenn & Sellbom, 2015; Muris et al., 2017). This is also evidenced through the construction and validation of psychopathy measures—the PPI-R includes the subscale measuring Machievellian Egocentricity (measuring both Machiavellianism and narcissism), while other measures of psychopathy directly (e.g., EPA) or indirectly measure narcissism (e.g., PCL R criterion *grandiose sense of self-worth*). While the Dark Triad is a popular and captivating way of conceptualizing what hides in the dark corners of malevolent human behavior, it appears to have further complicated the long-standing conceptual debate surrounding psychopathy.

2.6 Chapter Conclusion

Sparked by Cleckley (1941) and fueled by the empirical work of Hare and his research team (1980), the conceptualization of psychopathy has been afforded a tremendous amount of critical thought and examination by a multitude of researchers across a host of countries and populations. Decades of theorizing and scientific inquiry led to a multitude of conceptualizations and measurements of psychopathy, including, but not limited to the PCL/PCL-R, LSRP, PPI/PPI-R, TriPM, EPA, and the Dark Triad. Although the conceptualizations share many overlapping features, such as the tendency for psychopaths to behave in socially aversive ways, there is no unequivocal agreement on what traits and behaviors define the construct. While the literature has succeeded at providing an incredibly informed, nuanced, and scientific perspective on the construct, a cloud of confusion lurks in the shadows of these achievements. Although there is cumulative strong evidence for the dimensional nature of psychopathy, less clarity surrounds the role of antisociality and arguably adaptive traits and unanimity over the fundamental features of the construct remains elusive.

Thus, there is not one best way to describe or recognize a psychopath—at least, not without the risk of failure to give due credit to certain traits (e.g., adaptive features, antisociality). While affording full respect to Hare's work (1991, 2003) in the conceptualization psychopathy, given the diverse empirical advances in this context, individuals who risk contact with psychopaths (i.e., anyone who engages in social interaction) may find it prudent to consider the value of *all* conceptualizations of psychopathy rather than marrying themselves to one understanding or measure. Otherwise, they might find themselves caught unaware (or perhaps even worse) by deleterious commanders of psychopathic traits.

References

Ackerman, R. A., Witt, E. A., Donnellan, M. B., Trzesniewski, K. H., Robins, R. W., & Kashy, D. A. (2011). What does the narcissistic personality inventory really measure? *Assessment, 18*(1), 67–87. https://doi.org/10.1177/1073191110382845

Andershed, H., Kerr, M., Stattin, H., & Levander, S. (2002). Psychopathic traits in non-referred youths: Initial test of a new assessment tool. In E. Blaauw & L. Sheridan (Eds.), *Psychopaths: Current international perspectives* (pp. 131–158). Elsevier.

Anderson, J. L., Sellbom, M., Wygant, D. B., & Edens, J. F. (2013). Examining the necessity for and utility of the Psychopathic Personality Inventory—Revised (PPI-R) validity scales. *Law and Human Behavior, 37*(5), 312–320. https://doi.org/10.1037/lhb0000018

Anestis, J. C., Caron, K. M., & Carbonell, J. L. (2011). Examining the impact of gender on the factor structure of the psychopathic personality inventory – Revised. *Assessment, 18*(3), 340–349. https://doi.org/10.1007/s10862-017-9588-8

Babiak, P., Neumann, C. S., & Hare, R. D. (2010). Corporate psychopathy: Talking the walk. *Behavioral Sciences & the Law, 28*(2), 174–193. https://doi.org/10.1002/bsl.925

Benning, S. D., Patrick, C. J., Hicks, B. M., Blonigen, D. M., & Krueger, R. F. (2003). Factor structure of the psychopathic personality inventory: Validity and implications for clinical assessment. *Psychological Assessment, 15*(3), 340–350. https://doi.org/10.1037/1040-3590.15.3.340

Benning, S. D., Patrick, C. J., Salekin, R. T., & Leistico, A. M. R. (2005). Convergent and discriminant validity of psychopathy factors assessed via self-report: A comparison of three instruments. *Assessment, 12*(3), 270–289. https://doi.org/10.1177/1073191105277110

Benning, S. D., Venables, N. C., & Hall, J. R. (2018). Successful psychopathy. In C. J. Patrick (Ed.), *Handbook of psychopathy* (2nd ed., pp. 585–608). The Guilford Press.

Berardino, S. D., Meloy, J. R., Sherman, M., & Jacobs, D. (2005). Validation of the psychopathic personality inventory on a female inmate sample. *Behavioral Sciences & the Law, 23*(6), 819–836. https://doi.org/10.1002/bsl.666

Berg, J. M., Hecht, L. K., Latzman, R. D., & Lilienfeld, S. O. (2015). Examining the correlates of the coldheartedness factor of the psychopathic personality inventory – Revised. *Psychological Assessment, 27*(4), 1494–1499. https://doi.org/10.1037/pas0000129

Berg, J. M., Lilienfeld, S. O., & Sellbom, M. (2017). The role of boldness in psychopathy: A study of academic and clinical perceptions. *Personality Disorders: Theory, Research, and Treatment, 8*(4), 319–328. https://doi.org/10.1037/per0000247

Blagov, P. S., Patrick, C. J., Oost, K. M., Goodman, J. A., & Pugh, A. T. (2016). Triarchic psychopathy measure: Validity in relation to normal-range traits, personality pathology, and psychological adjustment. *Journal of Personality Disorders, 30*(1), 71–81. https://doi.org/10.1521/pedi_2015_29_182

Brinkley, C. A., Diamond, P. M., Magaletta, P. R., & Heigel, C. P. (2008). Cross-validation of Levenson's psychopathy scale in a sample of federal female inmates. *Assessment, 15*(4), 464–482. https://doi.org/10.1177/1073191108319043

Brown, R. P., Budzek, K., & Tamborski, M. (2009). On the meaning and measure of narcissism. *Personality and Social Psychology Bulletin, 35*(7), 951–964. https://doi.org/10.1177/0146167209335461

Campbell, D. T., & Fiske, D. W. (1959). Convergent and discriminant validation by the multitrait-multimethod matrix. *Psychological Bulletin, 56*(2), 81–105. https://doi.org/10.1037/h0046016

Christian, E., & Sellbom, M. (2016). Development and validation of an expanded version of the three-factor Levenson self-report psychopathy scale. *Journal of Personality Assessment, 98*(2), 155–168. https://doi.org/10.1080/00223891.2015.1068176

Christie, R., & Geis, F. L. (1970). *Studies in Machiavellianism*. Academic.

Cleckley, H. (1941). *The mask of sanity*. Mosby.

Cleckley, H. (1976). *The mask of sanity* (5th ed.). Mosby.

Collison, K. L., Miller, J. D., & Lynam, D. R. (2021). Examining the factor structure and valid-
    ity of the triarchic model of psychopathy across measures. *Personality Disorders: Theory,
    Research, and Treatment, 12*(2), 115–126. https://doi.org/10.1037/per0000394
Cooke, D. J., & Michie, C. (2001). Refining the construct of psychopathy: Towards a hierarchical
    model. *Psychological Assessment, 13*, 171–188. https://doi.org/10.1037/1040-3590.13.2.171
Costa, P. T., Jr., & McCrae, R. R. (1992). *Revised NEO Personality Inventory (NEO-PI–R) and
    NEO Five-Factor Inventory (NEO-FFI) professional manual.* Psychological Assessment
    Resources.
Crego, C., & Widiger, T. A. (2014). Psychopathy, DSM-5, and a caution. *Personality Disorders:
    Theory, Research, and Treatment, 5*(4), 335–347. https://doi.org/10.1037/per0000078
Crowe, M. L., Weiss, B. M., Sleep, C. E., Harris, A. M., Carter, N. T., Lynam, D. R., & Miller,
    J. D. (2021). Fearless dominance/boldness is not strongly related to externalizing behaviors:
    An item response-based analysis. *Assessment, 28*(2), 413–428.
Dolan, M., & Doyle, M. (2000). Violence risk prediction: Clinical and actuarial measures and the
    role of the psychopathy checklist. *The British Journal of Psychiatry, 177*(4), 303–311. https://
    doi.org/10.1192/bjp.177.4.303
Drislane, L. E., & Patrick, C. J. (2017). Integrating alternative conceptions of psychopathic per-
    sonality: A latent variable model of triarchic psychopathy constructs. *Journal of personality
    disorders, 31*(1), 110–132. https://doi.org/10.1521/pedi_2016_30_240
Edens, J. F., & McDermott, B. E. (2010). Examining the construct validity of the psychopathic
    personality inventory–revised: Preferential correlates of fearless dominance and self-centered
    impulsivity. *Psychological Assessment, 22*(1), 32–42. https://doi.org/10.1037/a0018220
Eichenbaum, A. E., Marcus, D. K., & French, B. F. (2021). Item response theory analysis of the
    triarchic psychopathy measure. *Psychological Assessment.* Advance online publication. https://
    doi.org/10.1037/pas0001022
Fanti, K. A., Lordos, A., Sullivan, E. A., & Kosson, D. S. (2018). Cultural and ethnic variations
    in psychopathy. In C. J. Patrick (Ed.), *Handbook of psychopathy* (2nd ed., pp. 529–569). The
    Guilford Press.
Few, L. R., Miller, J. D., & Lynam, D. R. (2013). An examination of the factor structure of the
    elemental psychopathy assessment. *Personality Disorders: Theory, Research, and Treatment,
    4*(3), 247–253. https://doi.org/10.1037/per0000016
Forth, A. E., Hart, S. D., & Hare, R. D. (1990). Assessment of psychopathy in male young
    offenders. *Psychological Assessment: A Journal of Consulting and Clinical Psychology, 2*(3),
    342–344. https://doi.org/10.1037/1040-3590.2.3.342
Forth, A. E., Brown, S. L., Hart, S. D., & Hare, R. D. (1996). The assessment of psychopathy in
    male and female noncriminals: Reliability and validity. *Personality and Individual Differences,
    20*, 531–543. https://doi.org/10.1016/0191-8869(95)00221-9
Frick, P. J., & Hare, R. D. (2001). *Antisocial process screening device (APSD): Technical manual.*
    Multi Health Systems.
Glenn, A. L., & Sellbom, M. (2015). Theoretical and empirical concerns regarding the Dark Triad
    as a construct. *Journal of Personality Disorders, 29*(3), 360–377. https://doi.org/10.1521/
    pedi_2014_28_162
Goodboy, A. K., & Martin, M. M. (2015). The personality profile of a cyberbully: Examining the
    dark triad. *Computers in Human Behavior, 49*, 1–4. https://doi.org/10.1016/j.chb.2015.02.052
Guay, J. P., Ruscio, J., Knight, R. A., & Hare, R. D. (2007). A taxometric analysis of the latent
    structure of psychopathy: Evidence for dimensionality. *Journal of Abnormal Psychology,
    116*(4), 701–716. https://doi.org/10.1037/0021-843X.116.4.701
Hall, J. R., Benning, S. D., & Patrick, C. J. (2004). Criterion-related validity of the three-factor
    model of psychopathy: Personality, behavior, and adaptive functioning. *Assessment, 11*(1),
    4–16. https://doi.org/10.1177/1073191103261466
Hare, R. D. (1980). A research scale for the assessment of psychopathy in crimi-
    nal populations. *Personality and Individual Differences, 1*, 111–119. https://doi.
    org/10.1016/0191-8869(80)90028-8

Hare, R. D. (1985). Comparison of procedures for the assessment of psychopathy. *Journal of Consulting and Clinical Psychology, 53*(1), 7–16. https://doi.org/10.1037/0022-006X.53.1.7

Hare, R. D. (1991). *The Hare psychopathy checklist – Revised*. Multi Health Systems.

Hare, R. D. (2003). *The Hare psychopathy checklist – Revised* (2nd ed.). Multi-Health Systems.

Hare, R. D. (2021). The PCL-R assessment of psychopathy. In A. R. Felthous & H. Saß (Eds.), *The Wiley International handbook on psychopathic disorders and the law* (2nd ed., pp. 63–106). Wiley.

Hare, R. D., & Neumann, C. S. (2008). Psychopathy as a clinical and empirical construct. *Annual Review of Clinical Psychology, 4*, 217–241. https://doi.org/10.1146/annurev.clinpsy.3.022806.091452

Hare, R. D., & Neumann, C. S. (2010). The role of antisociality in the psychopathy construct: Comment on Skeem and Cooke (2010). *Psychological Assessment, 22*(2), 446–454. https://doi.org/10.1037/a0013635

Hare, R. D., Harpur, T. J., Hakstian, A. R., Forth, A. E., Hart, S. D., & Newman, J. P. (1990). The revised psychopathy checklist: Reliability and factor structure. *Psychological Assessment: A Journal of Consulting and Clinical Psychology, 2*(3), 338–341.

Harpur, T. J., Hakstian, A. R., & Hare, R. D. (1988). Factor structure of the psychopathy checklist. *Journal of Consulting and Clinical Psychology, 56*, 741–747.

Harpur, T. J., Hare, R., & Hakstian, A. R. (1989). Two-factor conceptualization of psychopathy: Construct validity and assessment implications. *Psychological Assessment, 1*, 6–17.

John, O. P., Donahue, E. M., & Kentle, R. L. (1991). *The big five inventory-versions 4a and 54*. University of California, Berkeley, Institute of Personality and Social Research.

Jonason, P. K. (2015). How "dark" personality traits and perceptions come together to predict racism in Australia. *Personality and Individual Differences, 72*, 47–51. https://doi.org/10.1016/j.paid.2014.08.030

Jonason, P. K., & Webster, G. D. (2010). The dirty dozen: A concise measure of the dark triad. *Psychological Assessment, 22*, 420–432. https://doi.org/10.1037/a0019265

Jones, D. N. (2014). Risk in the face of retribution: Psychopathic individuals persist in financial misbehavior among the dark triad. *Personality and Individual Differences, 67*, 109–113.

Jones, D. N., & Paulhus, D. L. (2014). Introducing the Short Dark Triad (SD3): A brief measure of dark personality traits. *Assessment, 21*, 28–41. https://doi.org/10.1177/1073191113514105

Karpman, B. (1948). The myth of psychopathic personality. *American Journal of Psychiatry, 103*, 523–534.

Khiroya, R., Weaver, T., & Maden, T. (2009). Use and perceived utility of structured violence risk assessments in English medium secure forensic units. *Psychiatric Bulletin, 33*(4), 129–132. https://doi.org/10.1192/pb.bp.108.019810

Krueger, R. F., Markon, K. E., Patrick, C. J., Benning, S. D., & Kramer, M. D. (2007). Linking antisocial behavior, substance use, and personality: An integrative quantitative model of the adult externalizing spectrum. *Journal of Abnormal Psychology, 116*(4), 645–666. https://doi.org/10.1037/0021-843X.116.4.645

Kubarych, T. S., Deary, I. J., & Austin, E. J. (2004). The narcissistic personality inventory: Factor structure in a non-clinical sample. *Personality and Individual Differences, 36*(4), 857–872. https://doi.org/10.1016/S0191-8869(03)00158-2

Latzman, R. D., Palumbo, I. M., Sauvigné, K. C., Hecht, L. K., Lilienfeld, S. O., & Patrick, C. J. (2019). Psychopathy and internalizing psychopathology: A triarchic model perspective. *Journal of Personality Disorders, 33*(2), 262–287. https://doi.org/10.1521/pedi_2018_32_347

Levenson, M. R., Kiehl, K. A., & Fitzpatrick, C. M. (1995). Assessing psychopathic attributes in a noninstitutionalized population. *Journal of Personality and Social Psychology, 68*(1), 151–158. https://doi.org/10.1037/0022-3514.68.1.151

Lilienfeld, S. O. (2013). Is psychopathy a syndrome? Commentary on Marcus, Fulton, and Edens. *Personality Disorders: Theory, Research, and Treatment, 4*(1), 85–86. https://doi.org/10.1037/a0027544

Lilienfeld, S. O., & Andrews, B. P. (1996). Development and preliminary validation of a self-report measure of psychopathic personality traits in noncriminal population. *Journal of Personality Assessment, 66*(3), 488–524. https://doi.org/10.1207/s15327752jpa6603_3

Lilienfeld, S. O., & Fowler, K. A. (2006). The self-report assessment of psychopathy: Problems, pitfalls, and promises. In C. J. Patrick (Ed.), *Handbook of psychopathy* (2nd ed., pp. 107–132). The Guilford Press.

Lilienfeld, S. O., & Hess, T. H. (2001). Psychopathic personality traits and somatization: Sex differences and the mediating role of negative emotionality. *Journal of Psychopathology and Behavioral Assessment, 23*(1), 11–24. https://doi.org/10.1023/A:1011035306061

Lilienfeld, S. O., & Widows, M. (2005). *Psychopathic personality inventory – Revised professional manual*. Psychological Assessment Resources.

Lilienfeld, S. O., Patrick, C. J., Benning, S. D., Berg, J., Sellbom, M., & Edens, J. F. (2012). The role of fearless dominance in psychopathy: Confusions, controversies, and clarifications. *Personality Disorders: Theory, Research, and Treatment, 3*, 327–340. https://doi.org/10.1037/a0026987

Lilienfeld, S. O., Smith, S. F., Sauvigné, K. C., Patrick, C. J., Drislane, L. E., Latzman, R. D., & Krueger, R. F. (2016). Is boldness relevant to psychopathic personality? Meta-analytic relations with non-psychopathy checklist-based measures of psychopathy. *Psychological Assessment, 28*, 1172–1185. https://doi.org/10.1037/pas0000244

Lynam, D. R., & Widiger, T. A. (2007). Using a general model of personality to identify the basic elements of psychopathy. *Journal of Personality Disorders, 21*(2), 160–178. https://doi.org/10.1521/pedi.2007.21.2.160

Lynam, D. R., Whiteside, S., & Jones, S. (1999). Self-reported psychopathy: A validation study. *Journal of Personality Assessment, 73*(1), 110–132.

Lynam, D. R., Gaughan, E. T., Miller, J. D., Miller, D. J., Mullins-Sweatt, S., & Widiger, T. A. (2011). Assessing the basic traits associated with psychopathy: Development and validation of the elemental psychopathy assessment. *Psychological Assessment, 23*(1), 108–124. https://doi.org/10.1037/a0021146

Maheux-Caron, V., Gamache, D., Sellbom, M., Christian, E., Lussier, Y., & Savard, C. (2020). French adaptation and validation of the expanded version of the three-factor Levenson self-report psychopathy scale. *Assessment, 27*(7), 1448–1462. https://doi.org/10.1177/1073191118811607

Maples, J. L., Lamkin, J., & Miller, J. D. (2014). A test of two brief measures of the dark triad: The dirty dozen and the short dark triad. *Psychological Assessment, 26*, 326–331. https://doi.org/10.1037/a0035084

Marcus, D. K., Fulton, J. J., & Edens, J. F. (2013). The two-factor model of psychopathic personality: Evidence from the psychopathic personality inventory *Personality Disorders: Theory, Research, and Treatment, 4*(1), 67, 140–154. https://doi.org/10.1037/a0025282

McCrae, R. R., & Costa, P. T., Jr. (1990). *Personality in adulthood*. Guilford Press.

Miller, J. D., & Lynam, D. R. (2012). An examination of the psychopathic personality inventory's nomological network: A meta-analytic review. *Personality Disorders: Theory, Research, and Treatment, 3*(3), 305–326. https://doi.org/10.1037/a0024567

Miller, J. D., & Lynam, D. R. (2015). Understanding psychopathy using the basic elements of personality. *Social and Personality Psychology Compass, 9*(5), 223–237. https://doi.org/10.1111/spc3.12170

Miller, J. D., Lynam, D. R., Widiger, T. A., & Leukefeld, C. (2001). Personality disorders as extreme variants of common personality dimensions: Can the five-factor model adequately represent psychopathy? *Journal of Personality, 69*(2), 253–276. https://doi.org/10.1111/1467-6494.00144

Miller, J. D., Gaughan, E. T., Maples, J., Gentile, B., Lynam, D. R., & Widiger, T. A. (2011a). Examining the construct validity of the elemental psychopathy assessment. *Assessment, 18*, 106–114. https://doi.org/10.1177/1073191110393139

Miller, J. D., Jones, S. E., & Lynam, D. R. (2011b). Psychopathic traits from the perspective of self and informant reports: Is there evidence for a lack of insight? *Journal of Abnormal Psychology, 120*, 758–764. https://doi.org/10.1037/a0022477

Miller, J. D., Few, L. R., Seibert, L. A., Watts, A., Zeichner, A., & Lynam, D. R. (2012). An examination of the dirty dozen measure of psychopathy: A cautionary tale about the costs of brief measures. *Psychological Assessment, 24*(4), 1048–1053. https://doi.org/10.1037/a0028583

Miller, J. D., Hyatt, C. S., Rausher, S., Maples, J. L., & Zeichner, A. (2014). A test of the construct validity of the elemental psychopathy assessment scores in a community sample of adults. *Psychological Assessment, 26*(2), 555–562. https://doi.org/10.1037/a0035952

Muris, P., Merckelbach, H., Otgaar, H., & Meijer, E. (2017). The malevolent side of human nature: A meta-analysis and critical review of the literature on the dark triad (narcissism, Machiavellianism, and psychopathy). *Perspectives on Psychological Science, 12*(2), 183–204. https://doi.org/10.1177/1745691616666070

Neumann, C. S., Hare, R. D., & Newman, J. P. (2007). The super-ordinate nature of the psychopathy checklist-revised. *Journal of Personality Disorders, 21*(2), 102–117. https://doi.org/10.1521/pedi.2007.21.2.102

Neumann, C. S., Hare, R. D., & Pardini, D. A. (2015). Antisociality and the construct of psychopathy: Data from across the globe. *Journal of Personality, 83*, 678–692. https://doi.org/10.1111/jopy.12127

Neumann, C. S., Malterer, M. B., & Newman, J. P. (2008). Factor structure of the Psychopathic Personality Inventory (PPI): Findings from a large incarcerated sample. *Psychological Assessment, 20*(2), 169–174. https://doi.org/10.1037/1040-3590.20.2.169

Patrick, C. J. (2010). *Operationalising the Triarchic conceptualisation of psychopathy: Preliminary description of brief scales for assessment of boldness.* Meanness and Disinhibition. Unpublished manual, Florida State University.

Patrick, C. J., Fowles, D. C., & Krueger, R. F. (2009). Triarchic conceptualization of psychopathy: Developmental origins of disinhibition, boldness, and meanness. *Development and Psychopathology, 21*(3), 913–938. https://doi.org/10.1017/S0954579409000492

Patrick, C. J., Drislane, L. E., & Strickland, C. (2012). Conceptualizing psychopathy in triarchic terms: Implications for treatment. *International Journal of Forensic Mental Health, 11*(4), 253–266. https://doi.org/10.1080/14999013.2012.746761

Patrick, C. J., Venables, N. C., & Drislane, L. E. (2013). The role of fearless dominance in differentiating psychopathy from antisocial personality disorder: Comment on Marcus, Fulton, and Edens. *Personality Disorders: Theory, Research, and Treatment, 4*(1), 80–82. https://doi.org/10.1037/a0027173

Paulhus, D. L., & Williams, K. M. (2002). The dark triad of personality: Narcissism, Machiavellianism, and psychopathy. *Journal of Research in Personality, 36*(6), 556–563. https://doi.org/10.1016/S0092-6566(02)00505-6

Paulhus, D. L., Neumann, C. S., & Hare, R. D. (2016). *Manual for the self-report psychopathy scale.* Multi-Health Systems.

Poythress, N. G., Edens, J. F., & Lilienfeld, S. O. (1998). Criterion-related validity of the psychopathic personality inventory in a prison sample. *Psychological Assessment, 10*(4), 426–430. https://doi.org/10.1037/1040-3590.10.4.426

Poythress, N. G., Lilienfeld, S. O., Skeem, J. L., Douglas, K. S., Edens, J. F., Epstein, M., & Patrick, C. J. (2010). Using the PCL-R to help estimate the validity of two self-report measures of psychopathy with offenders. *Assessment, 17*(2), 206–219. https://doi.org/10.1177/1073191109351715

Quinsey, V. L., Rice, M. E., & Harris, G. T. (1995). Actuarial prediction of sexual recidivism. *Journal of Interpersonal Violence, 10*(1), 85–105. https://doi.org/10.1177/088626095010001006

Raskin, R., & Hall, C. S. (1979). A narcissistic personality inventory. *Psychological Reports, 45*, 590. https://doi.org/10.2466/pr0.1979.45.2.590

Raskin, R., & Terry, H. (1988). A principal-components analysis of the narcissistic personality inventory and further evidence of its construct validity. *Journal of Personality and Social Psychology, 54*, 890–902. https://doi.org/10.1037/0022-3514.54.5.890

Ray, J. V., Hall, J., Rivera-Hudson, N., Poythress, N. G., Lilienfeld, S. O., & Morano, M. (2013). The relation between self-reported psychopathic traits and distorted response styles: A meta-analytic review. *Personality Disorders: Theory, Research, and Treatment, 4*, 1–14. https://doi.org/10.1037/a0026482

Ross, S. R., Benning, S. D., Patrick, C. J., Thompson, A., & Thurston, A. (2009). Factors of the psychopathic personality inventory: Criterion-related validity and relationship to the BIS/BAS and five-factor models of personality. *Assessment, 16*(1), 71–87. https://doi.org/10.1177/1073191108322207

Roy, S., Vize, C., Uzieblo, K., van Dongen, J. D. M., Miller, J., Lynam, D., Brazil, I., Yoon, D., Mokros, A., Gray, N. S., Snowden, R., & Neumann, C. S. (2021). Triarchic or septarchic? -uncovering the Triarchic Psychopathy Measure's (TriPM) structure. *Personality Disorders: Theory, Research, and Treatment, 12*(1), 1–15. https://doi.org/10.1037/per0000392

Ruchensky, J. R., Edens, J. F., Corker, K. S., Donnellan, M. B., Witt, E. A., & Blonigen, D. M. (2018). Evaluating the structure of psychopathic personality traits: A meta-analysis of the psychopathic personality inventory. *Psychological Assessment, 30*(6), 707–718. https://doi.org/10.1037/pas0000520

Salekin, R. T., Rogers, R., & Sewell, K. W. (1996). A review and meta-analysis of the psychopathy checklist and psychopathy checklist-revised: Predictive validity of dangerousness. *Clinical Psychology: Science and Practice, 3*(3), 203–215. https://doi.org/10.1111/j.1468-2850.1996.tb00071.x

Salekin, R. T., Chen, D. R., Sellbom, M., Lester, W. S., & MacDougall, E. (2014). Examining the factor structure and convergent and discriminant validity of the Levenson self-report psychopathy scale: Is the two-factor model the best fitting model? *Personality Disorders: Theory, Research, and Treatment, 5*(3), 289–304. https://doi.org/10.1037/per0000073

Seibert, L. A., Miller, J. D., Few, L. R., Zeichner, A., & Lynam, D. R. (2011). An examination of the structure of self-report psychopathy measures and their relations with general traits and externalizing behaviors. *Personality Disorders: Theory, Research, and Treatment, 2*(3), 193–208. https://doi.org/10.1037/a0019232

Sellbom, M. (2011). Elaborating on the construct validity of the Levenson self-report psychopathy scale in incarcerated and non-incarcerated samples. *Law and Human Behavior, 35*(6), 440–451. https://doi.org/10.1007/s10979-010-9249-x

Sellbom, M., & Phillips, T. R. (2013). An examination of the triarchic conceptualization of psychopathy in incarcerated and nonincarcerated samples. *Journal of Abnormal Psychology, 122*(1), 208–214. https://doi.org/10.1037/a0029306

Sellbom, M., Lilienfeld, S. O., Fowler, K. A., & McCrary, K. L. (2018). The self-report assessment of psychopathy: Challenges, pitfalls, and promises. In C. J. Patrick (Ed.), *Handbook of psychopathy* (2nd ed., pp. 211–258). The Guilford Press.

Shou, Y., Sellbom, M., & Han, J. (2016). Development and validation of the Chinese Triarchic psychopathy measure. *Journal of Personality Disorders, 30*(4), 436–450. https://doi.org/10.1521/pedi.2016.30.4.436

Shou, Y., Sellbom, M., & Xu, J. (2018). Psychometric properties of the triarchic psychopathy measure: An item response theory approach. *Personality Disorders: Theory, Research, and Treatment, 9*(3), 217–227. https://doi.org/10.1037/per0000241

Skeem, J. L., & Cooke, D. J. (2010). Is criminal behavior a central component of psychopathy? Conceptual directions for resolving the debate. *Psychological Assessment, 22*, 433–445. https://doi.org/10.1037/a0008512

Skeem, J. L., Mulvey, E. P., & Grisso, T. (2003). Applicability of traditional and revised models of psychopathy to the psychopathy checklist: Screening version. *Psychological Assessment, 15*(1), 41–55. https://doi.org/10.1037/1040-3590.15.1.41

Somma, A., Fossati, A., Patrick, C., Maffei, C., & Borroni, S. (2014). The three-factor structure of the Levenson self-report psychopathy scale: Fool's gold or true gold? A study in a sample of Italian adult non-clinical participants. *Personality and Mental Health, 8*(4), 337–347. https://doi.org/10.1002/pmh.1267

Somma, A., Borroni, S., Drislane, L. E., Patrick, C. J., & Fossati, A. (2019). Modeling the structure of the triarchic psychopathy measure: Conceptual, empirical, and analytic considerations. *Journal of Personality Disorders, 33*(4), 470–496. https://doi.org/10.1521/pedi_2018_32_354

Stanley, J. H., Wygant, D. B., & Sellbom, M. (2013). Elaborating on the construct validity of the triarchic psychopathy measure in a criminal offender sample. *Journal of Personality Assessment, 95*(4), 343–350. https://doi.org/10.1080/00223891.2012.735302

Stanton, K., Brown, M. F. D., & Watson, D. (2021). Examining the item-level structure of the triarchic psychopathy measure: Sharpening assessment of psychopathy constructs. *Assessment, 28*(2), 429–445. https://doi.org/10.1177/1073191120927786

Vitacco, M. J., Neumann, C. S., & Jackson, R. L. (2005). Testing a four-factor model of psychopathy and its association with ethnicity, gender, intelligence, and violence. *Journal of Consulting and Clinical Psychology, 73*(3), 466–476. https://doi.org/10.1037/0022-006X.73.3.466

Wall, T. D., Wygant, D. B., & Sellbom, M. (2015). Boldness explains a key difference between psychopathy and antisocial personality disorder. *Psychiatry, Psychology and Law, 22*(1), 94–105. https://doi.org/10.1080/13218719.2014.919627

Widiger, T. A., & Lynam, D. R. (1998). Psychopathy and the five-factor model of personality. In T. Millon, E. Simonsen, M. Birket-Smith, & R. D. Davis (Eds.), *Psychopathy: Antisocial, criminal, and violent behavior* (pp. 171–187). The Guilford Press.

Wilson, L., Miller, J. D., Zeichner, A., Lynam, D. R., & Widiger, T. A. (2011). An examination of the validity of the elemental psychopathy assessment: Relations with other psychopathy measures, aggression, and externalizing behaviors. *Journal of Psychopathology and Behavioral Assessment, 33*, 315–322. https://doi.org/10.1007/s10862-010-9213-6

Witt, E. A., Donnellan, M. B., & Blonigen, D. M. (2009a). Using existing self-report inventories to measure the psychopathic personality traits of fearless dominance and impulsive antisociality. *Journal of Research in Personality, 43*(6), 1006–1016. https://doi.org/10.1016/j.jrp.2009.06.010

Witt, E. A., Donnellan, M. B., Blonigen, D. M., Krueger, R. F., & Conger, R. D. (2009b). Assessment of fearless dominance and impulsive antisociality via normal personality measures: Convergent validity, criterion validity, and developmental change. *Journal of Personality Assessment, 91*(3), 265–276. https://doi.org/10.1080/00223890902794317

Chapter 3
Health Professions

3.1 Introduction

As a high-risk population (Reidy et al., 2015), individuals with psychopathic traits are often found within a medical setting. Whether that is as patients or as medical professionals, it is likely that individuals with psychopathic traits will be encountered by those in the healthcare field. Psychopathic traits are considered a risk factor for severe and chronic violence and contribute to a large burden on the public health and criminal justice systems (Reidy et al., 2015). Violence can lead not only to physical injuries but also may have long-term medical and mental impacts. Reidy et al. (2015) suggest that the public health approach to violence has generally neglected to consider this key variable and that the public health approach to violence prevention is focused on achieving change at the population level rather than the individual level. Increasing attention to the individual-level factor of psychopathy, focusing on primary prevention, and measuring psychopathy in public health research may improve the ability to prevent violence at the community and societal levels (Reidy et al., 2015).

Understanding the concept of psychopathy within a medical setting and recognizing common presentations of psychopathic traits are important concepts for health professionals covered in this chapter. Patients with psychopathic traits may require more mental and physical effort from medical professionals to effectively assess, treat, and manage. Additionally, common misconceptions regarding the treatment of psychopathic traits are explored. Preliminary evidence suggests that future interventions may focus on developmental considerations and neurobiological correlates of psychopathic traits. In contrast, traits of a "successful" psychopath may be found within clinical professions, and it is important to understand these individuals as well. These traits may be adaptive in medical professionals, providing additional protection against workplace stressors.

T. D. Kennedy et al., *Working with Psychopathy*, SpringerBriefs in Psychology, https://doi.org/10.1007/978-3-030-84025-9_3

3.2   Psychopathy in the DSM

Clinically, psychopathy is a confusing construct that is difficult to define. Psychopathy is not a disorder found in the current Diagnostic and Statistical Manual of Mental Disorders (DSM-5). Healthcare professionals are not provided with a formal indicator of psychopathy in patient charts or medical history. As a formal diagnosis, antisocial personality disorder is the only available diagnosis for clinicians to loosely identify a psychopath. Throughout the different versions of the DSM, psychopathy and psychopathic traits have evolved as a diagnosis. In the DSM-I, "sociopathic personality disturbance" with a specifier that included "antisocial reaction" based on Cleckley's definition of psychopathy was included (Crego & Widiger, 2015). This definition became more specific in the DSM-II, which included an "antisocial personality" that was expanded from the DSM-I and specified that a history of criminality is not sufficient as justification for this diagnosis (Crego & Widiger, 2015). From there, in the DSM-III, antisocial personality disorder provided a diagnosis for psychopathy. The criteria for this disorder were not based on Cleckley's definition, but rather distinguished offenders from nonoffenders through the inclusion of antisocial behaviors (Stevens, 1994). In the DSM-III-R, antisocial personality disorder relied on assessing for behaviors rather than examining personality traits as well as behaviors like those found in the PCL (Crego & Widiger, 2015). The DSM-IV further established specific criteria for antisocial personality disorder based on Factor 2 of the PCL-R, including adult criminal behavior (Crego & Widiger, 2015). These criteria paved the way for the current DSM-5, which includes the maladaptive traits that comprise antisocial personality disorder. A hybrid model of personality disorders was introduced, suggesting that future editions of the DSM include the triarchic model of psychopathy. This model includes recurring themes and identifies constructs like boldness, meanness, and disinhibition that are essential in the definition of psychopathy (Crego & Widiger, 2015).

3.3   Psychopathy Versus Antisocial Personality Disorder

Often, antisocial personality disorder has been used interchangeably with psychopathy, although there are clear differences between the two. In the DSM-5 alternative model of personality disorders, a dimensional, trait-based approach of antisocial personality disorder is considered, with the inclusion of impairment and maladaptive personality traits (Wygant et al., 2016). This conceptualization better predicts PCL-R scores in a male correctional sample (Wygant et al., 2016) and provides a distinctive diagnosis that better includes psychopathic traits. Until this expanded diagnostic option is available in the DSM-5, Ogloff (2006) suggests that research and clinical implications defined by the PCL-R should not be applied to diagnoses of antisocial personality disorder and dissocial personality disorder.

Despite the differences between antisocial personality disorder and psychopathy, many clinicians and researchers continue to use these terms interchangeably. For clinicians in a correctional setting, Stevens (1994) found that a minority of clinicians use the diagnosis of antisocial personality disorder and do not rely solely on the DSM criteria for diagnosis. These clinicians often diagnosed antisocial personality disorder using common characteristics of psychopathy and described those with this diagnosis as disruptive, manipulative, and hard to treat (Stevens, 1994). The common misuse of these terminologies may not only contribute to confusing and inconsistent research but also life-altering consequences for individuals who have been mislabeled. In a medical and psychological setting, clinicians typically utilize diagnostic criteria to inform effective treatment strategies for their patients. If the official diagnosis of antisocial personality disorder does not accurately capture the psychopathic symptoms of the patient, their treatment process could be negatively impacted.

3.4 Psychopathic Traits in Patients

Individuals with psychopathic personalities exist within the healthcare field. For those caring for these individuals, their valuable time and energy may be exhausted evaluating and managing these patients. Several studies have examined the characteristics and behaviors of these individuals in clinical settings. In a sample of 1026 participants in the waiting room of the medical emergency department of a city hospital, levels of fearless dominance similar to federal inmates were found (Benning et al., 2018). Fearless dominance is a concept included in the two- and three-factor models of psychopathy. It is often associated with less anxiety, depression, and empathy as well as increased functioning, assertiveness, and narcissism (Lilienfeld & Widows, 2005). In a medical emergency department, Fearless dominance was associated with agentic success (e.g., being employed, higher household income), fewer psychological problems, and less use of psychotropic medications (Benning et al., 2018). Because individuals with these traits may present as "successful," medical professionals may not be immediately aware of any psychopathic traits hidden beneath the surface. Further probing and observation may be necessary to complete the full picture of these individuals and their possible symptoms.

Additionally, levels of impulsive antisociality in patients from the waiting room of the medical emergency department were comparable to those of federal and state inmates (Benning et al., 2018). In this model of psychopathy, impulsive antisociality is associated with impulsivity, aggression, substance use, antisocial behavior, and suicidality (Lilienfeld & Widows, 2005). Impulsive antisociality was negatively related to both marital success and positively correlated with substance use and self-reported bipolar, ADHD, and psychotic psychiatric conditions (Benning et al., 2018). Further, impulsive antisociality was associated with presenting to the emergency department for physical injury or psychological disturbance (Benning et al., 2018). In patients with these characteristics, they are likely presenting to the medical department or emergency department with issues unrelated to any psycho-pathic traits. They may also be disruptive or aggressive, requiring extra attention from medical professionals to manage them. Fearless dominance and impulsive antisociality were both associated with male gender, younger age, and more fre-quent alcohol consumption (Benning et al., 2018). In an emergency department, personnel may want to be aware of these characteristics in patients, understanding that most individuals with psychopathic traits tend not to disclose psychopathy as a diagnosis or even be aware of exhibiting any of these characteristics. Instead, they may present to the emergency room with physical injuries, substance use, or other psychiatric conditions, while still demonstrating agentic success, depending on their specific psychopathic traits.

In psychiatric institutions and state hospitals, medical professions would likely encounter individuals with psychopathic traits. In an impatient setting, a disruptive patient could impact the environment and treatment for everyone on the unit. Jeandarme et al. (2017) found an association between psychopathy and therapy-interfering behavior (e.g., noncompliance, dropout, and misconduct). Individuals with these traits may be more likely to cause disruptions that affect the experience of other inpatients. As the general stress level of inpatients is significantly higher than a general population (Nigel et al., 2019), the added stressor of disruptive behavior from other patients could be especially upsetting. Comparatively, for those with psychopathic traits, psychological stress may not be as much of a concern. Utilizing the PPI-R, self-centered impulsivity was associated with high levels of stress, while fearless dominance was a negative predictor (Nigel et al., 2019). Fearless dominance could serve as a characteristic of resilience, protecting these individuals from stress symptoms in an inpatient unit. Despite lower levels of stress, individuals with psychopathic traits may not experience complete patient satisfac-tion. Dolan and Millington (2002) examined inpatients in a medium secure unit, where complainants among the forensic patients were compared to inpatients who had not made a complaint, to identify how psychopathy scores influenced the com-plaint procedure within this setting. Complainants had significantly higher PCL:SV scores and higher incident rates than non-complainants (Dolan & Millington, 2002). Specifically, "grandiosity" and "does not accept responsibility" significantly distin-guished complainants from non-complainants (Dolan & Millington, 2002). Staff and administration in forensic medical based settings should be aware of how per-sonality factors can impact patient satisfaction and complaints. Complaints require thorough investigation, including the circumstances surrounding the complaint and client satisfaction. Investigating these claims may distract healthcare professionals from providing essential care to other patients within the facility.

In a high security hospital, those in the dangerous and severe personality disorder (DSPD) units were compared with those in conventional medium or high security hospital units in the United Kingdom. Individuals in the DSPD had higher scores on the PCL-R, significantly more convictions before age 18 years, greater severity of institutional violence, and more prior crimes of sexual violence (Howard et al., 2012). PCL-R Factor 1, which includes core interpersonal and affective features of psychopathy, predicted group membership (Howard et al., 2012). In another study by Crocker et al. (2005), antisocial personality disorder, thought disturbance, negative affect, and earlier age at psychiatric hospitalization were predictive of aggressive behavior. It is important for clinicians and medical professionals to consider these differences and incorporate into the treatment and management of these individuals.

A common conception is that psychopathic traits are often associated with malingering or feigning mental disorders. The deceptive nature of psychopathic personalities suggests that manipulating clinicians is something that would be a common occurrence. Does the research really support this tendency? Poythress et al. (2001) examined this relationship and found that the association between the Psychopathic Personality Inventory (PPI) and malingering were not significant, suggesting that individuals with psychopathic traits were not more likely to fake symptoms of major mental illness.

3.5 Psychopathic Traits and Stigma

There is a clear stigma associated with the general public's understanding of a psychopath. There are common conceptions, and misconceptions, that many clinicians and medical professionals express. One shared idea is that individuals with psychopathic traits are difficult to treat. This therapeutic pessimism toward the treatment of psychopathic personalities may undermine motivation to search for effective modes of intervention for psychopathic individuals. Salekin (2002) examined the current literature on the treatment of psychopathy, which demonstrated little scientific basis for the belief that psychopathy is untreatable. Relevant research suggested that significant problems regarding the literature surrounding this topic include the inconsistent definition of psychopathy, the etiology of psychopathy, and the psychopathy-treatment relationship. Kirkman (2008) suggests that for forensic nurses (and doctors) working with psychopaths, a positive view about their own role and a therapeutic ward environment should be maintained.

Does Stigma Go Both Ways?
Do individuals with psychopathic characteristics hold the same stigmas as those without these traits? Durand et al. (2019) examined if individuals with psychopathic traits hold fewer stigmatizing beliefs toward this population. Six hundred and sixty-one participants from the community completed the Triarchic Psychopathy Measure and were randomly assigned to read a description of either a nonviolent or violent psychopath, as well as either a nonviolent or violent person with schizophrenia. Psychopathic traits were negatively associated with the stigmatization of individuals presented as either dangerous or non-dangerous psychopaths. These traits were not significantly associated with stigma toward schizophrenia or depression. Durand et al. (2019) suggested that this association may originate from feelings of similarity or from characteristics of fearlessness found in psychopathic personalities.

3.6   Interventions

In individuals with psychopathic traits, interventions are often a topic of contention among clinicians and researchers. In adolescents, results from treatment are often positive, providing hopeful evidence of treatment success (Salekin et al., 2010; Caldwell et al., 2006; Bailey et al., 2015). Adults with psychopathic traits, however, may not be as amenable to treatment. Outcomes of adults with psychopathic traits are mixed, suggesting inconsistencies in effectiveness. Although some studies suggest that interventions are not successful in individuals with psychopathic traits (Salekin et al., 2010), others provide evidence that specific treatments may result in positive outcomes (Skeem et al., 2002; Bailey et al., 2015; Pajerla & Felthous, 2007).

Individuals with psychopathic personality traits are often viewed by clinicians and researchers as resistant or immune to treatment. This concept has implications for individuals labeled "incurable," such as the effect of therapeutic pessimism on a clinical population. Although this perception is pervasive, it is important to understand and examine the literature surrounding treatment and psychopathic traits to encourage the future investigation of potential treatments. Salekin et al. (2010) examined research on the treatment of psychopathic traits. The articles they reviewed indicated that treatment in adults with psychopathic traits demonstrated low to moderate success. In contrast, Skeem et al. (2002) examined a sample of civil psychiatric patients and explored the association between psychopathy, the receipt of outpatient mental health services, and violence in the community. Results demonstrated that psychopathic patients were just a likely as non-psychopathic patients to benefit from adequate doses of treatment and a reduction in violence (Skeem et al., 2002). In a more recent review of the literature, Bailey et al. (2015) continued to find inconsistencies in treatment effectiveness. However, this review did find limited treatment effectiveness in cognitive behavioral therapy (CBT) and CBT-based treatments (Bailey et al., 2015). The recent application of these treatments may provide success in the treatment of behavioral traits of psychopathy. Pajerla and Felthous (2007) suggest that the identification of psychopathy may be useful in establishing an effective treatment context for common comorbid conditions, including substance abuse and aggression. By therapeutically addressing co-occurring conditions, clinicians can improve the patient's overall functioning even if they continue to exhibit psychopathic traits (Pajerla & Felthous, 2007). Although there is a strong foundation for the treatment resistance of psychopathic traits, promising alternatives may exist.

Despite any preliminary evidence of success in the treatment of psychopathic traits, a common conception is that treatment may make characteristics of psychopathy worse. D'Silva et al. (2004) evaluated the current literature on treatment responses of individuals with psychopathic traits. This review did not find sufficient evidence to support the theory that treatment may make psychopathic traits and behaviors worse, as only three studies fit their research design criteria and those three studies all held methodological flaws (D'Silva et al., 2004). Inconsistencies in the existing research can create consequences for individuals with psychopathic traits, as treatment pessimism and outright denial of treatment because of characteristics of an individual's personality provide a significant barrier to effective interventions.

In the treatment of youth with psychopathic traits, Salekin et al. (2010) found more promising results. Six of the eight studies they reviewed provided evidence of treatment benefits (Salekin et al., 2010). Caldwell et al. (2006) examined the treatment response of juvenile offenders with high scores on the Psychopathy Checklist: Youth Version (PCL: YV) who participated in an intensive treatment program or treatment as usual in a conventional juvenile correction institute. Offenders in the treatment as usual group were more than twice as likely to violently recidivate in the community during a 2-year follow-up than those who participated in intensive treatment (Caldwell et al., 2006). Additionally, this intensive treatment was associated with relatively slower and lower rates of serious recidivism (Caldwell et al., 2006). Multisystemic therapy also demonstrated effective results in the treatment of adolescent offenders with antisocial characteristics (Bailey et al., 2015). Results suggest that psychopathic traits in childhood and adolescence may be more amenable to treatment than in adulthood.

In recent literature, neurobiological correlates of psychopathic traits have become a relevant topic. In a study by Birbaumer et al. (2005), the functional magnetic resonance images of criminal psychopaths were compared to healthy control subjects. Compared to the general population, the cerebral, peripheral, and subjective correlates of fear conditioning in criminal psychopaths differed (Birbaumer et al., 2005). Psychopaths displayed no significant activity in emotional and cognitive processing areas of the brain (Birbaumer et al., 2005). Pickersgill (2011) suggests there is potential for neuroscience to contribute to clinical practice in the treatment of psychopathy. With further investigation into these correlates, these differences could potentially inform clinical practice in the examination and treatment of psychopathic traits.

3.7 Psychopathic Traits in Medical Professionals

As in many professions, occasionally those working in the medical field may exhibit psychopathic traits. Within the field of health professions, individuals holding different positions may exhibit psychopathic traits to different degrees. Bucknall et al. (2015) assessed the levels of "dark triad" personality traits, including psychopathy, in individuals working in different healthcare specialties. Healthcare professionals score significantly lower on psychopathy than the general population (Bucknall et al., 2015). Compared to other medical professionals, surgeons displayed a significantly higher level of primary psychopathy, while nursing professionals exhibited a significantly higher level of secondary psychopathy (Bucknall et al., 2015). In surgeons, primary psychopathic traits such as low anxiety and emotionality may be considered strengths in their high-stress career. Alternatively, for nursing professionals, secondary psychopathic traits, such as anxiety and neuroticism, may have developed because of job-related stress. Any neuroticism experienced by nurses could possibly lead to better patient care, as they pay even closer attention to detail. Overall, health professionals demonstrated lower levels of psychopathic traits than their patients. In the area of research and research misconduct, psychopathic traits are also found. Tijdink et al. (2016) examined the association between personality traits and self-reported questionable research practices and research misconduct in Dutch biomedical scientists. Psychopathic traits were found to be common in higher academic ranks, indicating that these traits may be desirable within the academic field (Tijdink et al., 2016). In encouraging responsible research behavior and academic administration, taking personality characteristics into account is an important consideration given the risk within this field.

Psychopathy is characterized by a lack of empathy for others. Clinical empathy describes the physician's ability to communicate his or her understanding of the emotional state of the patient. To avoid compassion fatigue and burnout, a decline of these capacities can be observed among physicians and medical students (Lemogne, 2015). To protect medical professionals from the negative effects of burnout, perspective-taking may be implemented to allow them to show sustained empathic concern while avoiding compassion fatigue (Lemogne, 2015). Possible interventions might be utilized to promote empathy among medical students before they begin patient care. These supportive services should target both communication skills and humanist values (Lemogne, 2015).

3.7.1   Dr. James Fallon (Stromberg, 2013)

Neuroscientist James Fallon, PhD, had dedicated his career to the study of neuroscience, including schizophrenia, Parkinson's disease, Alzheimer's disease, and addiction. In 2005, his research focused on the brain scans of serial killers and examining patterns in the brain associated with psychopathic traits. While looking at these scans, Dr. Fallon identified a scan that demonstrated low activity in areas of the frontal and temporal lobes connected with empathy and self-control, areas that are often impaired in individuals with psychopathic traits. When Dr. Fallon decided to look at the identity of this individual, he discovered that the scan belonged to him. He had submitted his own personal scans to research he was conducting on Alzheimer's disease but instead revealed his own psychopathic brain. After undergoing further genetic testing which indicated high-risk alleles for aggression, violence, and low empathy, Dr. Fallon reflected on his behavior and relationships in his life. Although he had never killed anyone or committed any crimes, Dr. Fallon reported that he had difficulties feeling true empathy for others, was motivated by power and manipulation, and found himself to be highly competitive. He believed that the positive environment in which he was raised prevented him from any violent or aggressive behavior, despite his genetic predisposition. Since this realization, Dr. Fallon has made efforts to change his behavior and consider others' feelings, although it does not come natural to him. He has since published a book on his experiences titled *The Psychopath Inside* and has shared his story in countless interviews to demonstrate inconsistency in the concept of psychopathy and the role that the environment and genetics play in its presentation.

3.8 Summary

Psychopathic traits are considered a risk factor for severe and chronic violence and contribute to a large burden on the public health and criminal justice systems (Reidy et al., 2015). Due to this impact, understanding the concept of psychopathy within a medical setting is an important concept for health professionals. These traits in patients may include manipulation, impulsivity, and anxiety. Psychopathy can be a difficult concept to define and is often utilized interchangeably with a diagnosis of antisocial personality disorder found in the DSM-5. Because of the differences between these two concepts, the literature remains puzzling and inconsistent regarding the nature of psychopathy.

Within a medical setting, individuals with psychopathic traits may behave differently than their counterparts. Impulsive antisociality and physical injury in an emergency department (Benning et al., 2018), filing complaints on an impatient unit (Dolan & Millington, 2002), and violence and aggressive behavior (Howard et al., 2012; Crocker et al., 2005) are some examples of these distinct behaviors that medical professionals may experience. Additionally, therapeutic pessimism may be pervasive among professionals working with individuals with psychopathic traits. Although there is a strong foundation for the treatment resistance of psychopathic traits, promising alternatives may exist, and it is important for medical professionals to consider the possibility of therapy for psychopathic characteristics.

Along with psychopathic traits being present in patients within a medical setting, characteristics of a "successful" psychopath may be found within clinical professions. These traits may include a lack of empathy (Lemogne, 2015), research misconduct (Tijdink et al., 2016), and features of primary or secondary psychopathy (Bucknall et al., 2015). Some of these characteristics may be advantageous in medical professionals, providing some benefits in their high-stress professions. Additionally, specific interventions and preventative measures can be implemented to encourage communication skills and humanist values (Lemogne, 2015) in these medical professionals.

For individuals working in the medical field, understanding this high-risk population and recognizing common presentations of psychopathic traits are important not only to protect these professionals but also to encourage future research on this topic that contributes to a more consistent and preventative conceptualization of psychopathy.

References

Bailey, C., Sehgal, R., Coscia, A., & Shelton, D. (2015). Exploring treatment options for an allegedly "untreatable" disorder, psychopathy: An integrative literature review. In M. E. Fitzgerald (Ed.), *Psychopathy: Risk factors, behavioral symptoms and treatment options*. Nova Science Publishers. https://doi.org/10.1037/t01167-000

Benning, S. D., Molina, S. M., Dowgwillo, E. A., Patrick, C. J., Miller, K. F., & Storrow, A. B. (2018). Psychopathy in the medical emergency department. *Journal of Personality Disorders, 32*(4), 482–496. https://doi.org/10.1521/pedi_2017_31_308

Birbaumer, N., Veit, R., Lotze, M., Erb, M., Hermann, C., Grodd, W., & Flor, H. (2005). Deficient fear conditioning in psychopathy: A functional magnetic resonance imaging study. *Archives of General Psychiatry*. https://doi.org/10.1001/archpsyc.62.7.799

Bucknall, V., Burwaiss, S., MacDonald, D., Charles, K., & Clement, R. (2015). Mirror mirror on the ward, who's the most narcissistic of them all? Pathologic personality traits in health care. *Canadian Medical Association Journal, 187*(18), 1359–1363. https://doi.org/10.1503/cmaj.151135

Caldwell, M., Skeem, J., Salekin, R., & Rybroek, G. V. (2006). Treatment response of adolescent offenders with psychopathy features: A 2-year follow-up. *Criminal Justice and Behavior; Thousand Oaks, 33*(5), 571–596. https://doi.org/10.1177/0093854806288176

Crego, C., & Widiger, T. A. (2015). Psychopathy and the DSM. *Journal of Personality, 83*(6), 665–677. https://doi.org/10.1111/jopy.12115

Crocker, A. G., Mueser, K. T., Drake, R. E., Clark, R. E., McHugo, G. J., Ackerson, T. H., & Alterman, A. I. (2005). Antisocial personality, psychopathy, and violence in persons with dual disorders: A longitudinal analysis. *Criminal Justice and Behavior, 32*(4), 452–476. https://doi.org/10.1177/0093854805276407

D'Silva, K., Duggan, C., & McCarthy, L. (2004). Does treatment really make psychopaths worse? A review of the evidence. *Journal of personality disorders, 18*(2), 163–177. https://doi.org/10.1521/pedi.18.2.163.32775

Dolan, M., & Millington, J. (2002). The influence of personality traits such as psychopathy on detained patients using the NHS complaints procedure in forensic settings. *Personality and Individual Differences, 33*(6), 955–965.

Durand, G., Metcalfe, R., & Arbone, I.-S. (2019). Affinity between us: Examining how psychopathic traits influence the stigmatization of psychiatric disorders. *Personality Disorders, 10*(6), 551–556. https://doi.org/10.1037/per0000362

Howard, R., Khalifa, N., Duggan, C., & Lumsden, J. (2012). Are patients deemed "dangerous and severely personality disordered" different from other personality disordered patients detained in forensic settings? *Criminal Behaviour and Mental Health: CBMH; London, 22*(1), 65. https://doi.org/10.1002/cbm.827

Jeandarme, I., Pouls, C., Oei, T. I., & Bogaerts, S. (2017). Forensic psychiatric patients with comorbid psychopathy: Double trouble? *The International Journal of Forensic Mental Health, 16*(2), 149–160. https://doi.org/10.1080/14999013.2017.1286414

Kirkman, C. A. (2008). Psychopathy: A confusing clinical construct. *Journal of Forensic Nursing; Baltimore, 4*(1), 29–39.

Lemogne, C. (2015). Empathy and medicine. *Bulletin de l'Academie nationale de medecine, 199*(2–3), 241–252.

Lilienfeld, S. O., & Widows, M. R. (2005). *Psychopathic personality inventory-revised: Professional manual*. Psychological Assessment Resources.

Nigel, S. M., Streb, J., Leichauer, K., Hennig, B., Otte, S., Franke, I., Helms, E., Weierstall, R., & Dudeck, M. (2019). The role of psychopathic personality traits in current psychological and physiological subclinical stress levels of forensic inpatients: A path analysis. *The International Journal of Forensic Mental Health, 18*(2), 164–177. https://doi.org/10.1080/14999013.2018.1532973

Ogloff, J. R. P. (2006). Psychopathy/antisocial personality disorder conundrum. *Australian and New Zealand Journal of Psychiatry, 40*(6–7), 519–528. https://doi.org/10.1080/j.1440-1614.2006.01834.x

Pajerla, S., MD, & Felthous, A. R., MD. (2007). The Paradox of psychopathy. *Psychiatric Times, 24*(13). Retrieved from https://www.psychiatrictimes.com/view/paradox-psychopathy

Pickersgill, M. (2011). Promising' therapies: Neuroscience, clinical practice, and the treatment of psychopathy. *Sociology of Health & Illness, 33*(3), 448–464. https://doi.org/10.1111/j.1467-9566.2010.01286.x

Poythress, N. G., Edens, J. F., & Watkins, M. M. (2001). The relationship between psychopathic personality features and malingering symptoms of major mental illness. *Law and Human Behavior; Southport, 25*(6), 567–582.

Reidy, D. E., Kearns, M. C., DeGue, S., Lilienfeld, S. O., Massetti, G., & Kiehl, K. A. (2015). Why psychopathy matters: Implications for public health and violence prevention. *Aggression and Violent Behavior, 24*, 214–225. https://doi.org/10.1016/j.avb.2015.05.018

Salekin, R. T. (2002). Psychopathy and therapeutic pessimism: Clinical lore or clinical reality? *Clinical Psychology Review, 22*(1), 79–112. https://doi.org/10.1016/s0272-7358(01)00083-6

Salekin, R. T., Worley, C., & Grimes, R. D. (2010). Treatment of psychopathy: A review and brief introduction to the mental model approach for psychopathy. *Behavioral Sciences & the Law, 28*(2), 235–266. https://doi.org/10.1002/bsl.928

Skeem, J. L., Monahan, J., & Mulvey, E. P. (2002). Psychopathy, treatment involvement, and subsequent violence among civil psychiatric patients. *Law and Human Behavior, 26*(6), 577–603.

Stevens, G. F. (1994). Prison clinicians' perceptions of antisocial personality disorder as a formal diagnosis. *Journal of Offender Rehabilitation, 20*(3–4), 159–185. https://doi.org/10.1300/J076v20n03_10

Stromberg, J. (2013). The neuroscientist who discovered he was a psychopath. *Smithsonian Magazine*. Retrieved May 14, 2021, from https://www.smithsonianmag.com/science-nature/the-neuroscientist-who-discovered-he-was-a-psychopath-180947814/

Tijdink, J. K., Bouter, L. M., Veldkamp, C. L., van de Ven, M., Wicherts, J. M., & Smulders, Y. M. (2016). Personality traits are associated with research misbehavior in Dutch scientists: A cross-sectional study. *PLoS One, 11*(9). https://doi.org/10.1371/journal.pone.0163251

Wygant, D. B., Sellbom, M., Sleep, C. E., Wall, T. D., Applegate, K. C., Krueger, R. F., & Patrick, C. J. (2016). Examining the DSM–5 alternative personality disorder model operationalization of antisocial personality disorder and psychopathy in a male correctional sample. *Personality Disorders: Theory, Research, and Treatment, 7*(3), 229–239. https://doi.org/10.1037/per0000179

Chapter 4
Forensic

4.1 Introduction

Professionals in law-based occupations may be more likely to interact with individuals with psychopathic characteristics (Kiehl & Hoffman, 2011). These careers include, but are not limited to, police officers, corrections officers, lawyers, and judges.

Professionals in these fields can more effectively arrest, interrogate, convict, and defend these individuals with an understanding of the relevant research. Individuals with psychopathic personality traits have a disproportionate impact on the criminal justice system. Psychopaths are 20–25 times more likely than non-psychopaths to be in prison and four to eight times more likely to violently recidivate compared to non-psychopaths and are resistant to many forms of treatment (Kiehl & Hoffman, 2011). Law enforcement officers, judges, and lawyers will likely interact with individuals with psychopathic personalities as criminals, clients, or defendants. It is particularly important for these professionals to be aware of psychopathy and to learn how to effectively interact with individuals with psychopathic traits.

Additionally, there are recent investigations into "successful" psychopaths within various legal professions. For example, high-profile incidents within the United States have encouraged research examining psychopathic personality traits in police officers. In fact, some characteristics of psychopathy, such as fearless temperament, may be related to successful functioning in careers like law enforcement (Falkenbach et al., 2018a, b). Knowing how to identify psychopaths, the effects these individuals have within this system, and how to work with them effectively is important for those working in legal professions.

T. D. Kennedy et al., *Working with Psychopathy*, SpringerBriefs in Psychology,
https://doi.org/10.1007/978-3-030-84025-9_4

4.2   Prevalence

The prevalence of psychopaths within the criminal justice system is significant. Psychopathic personalities make up roughly 1% of the general male adult population, and they make up between 15 and 25% of the males incarcerated in North American prison systems (Kiehl & Hoffman, 2011). Compared to the general population, psychopathic personalities are far more likely to be found within the criminal justice system. Even compared to individuals with other risk factors for incarceration, psychopaths are much more likely to be in prison. For example, an individual with a substance abuse problem is nine times more likely to be in prison compared to the general population, while individuals with a psychopathic personality are between 15 and 25 times more likely (Kiehl & Hoffman, 2011). Psychopathic personalities are also much more likely to recidivate and be violent offenders. Sixty-two percent of the general male population is made up of violent offenders, but 78% of imprisoned psychopaths are there because of a violent offense (Kiehl & Hoffman, 2011).

This high prevalence of psychopathic personalities within the criminal justice system poses a safety risk as well as a financial strain on society. Psychopaths are responsible for approximately $460 billion per year in criminal social costs (Kiehl & Hoffman, 2011). These costs do not include individuals in psychiatric hospitals or treatment for victims, which would substantially increase this number. Even compared to other conditions associated with criminality (e.g., substance use and schizophrenia), the cost is significantly higher. Given the negative impact of individuals with psychopathic traits on society and taxpayers, reduction of recidivism is essential.

4.3   Presentation

The law typically uses Hare's clinical definition of a psychopathic personality, which includes both the affective (Factor 1) and behavioral (Factor 2) characteristics of psychopathy. The minimum score on Hare's PCL-R (Hare, 1991, 2003) is 0, and the maximum is 40, with psychopathy defined as a score of 30 or more. Factor 1 includes traits related to the interpersonal and affective deficits of psychopathy. These include shallow affect, superficial charm, manipulativeness, and lack of empathy. Factor 2 criteria includes antisocial behavior associated with individuals who score high on the PCL-R. These behaviors are often driven by their desire for stimulation and their impulsive drive, including sexual promiscuity, impulsivity, irresponsibility, poor behavioral controls, juvenile delinquency, criminal versatility, and a parasitic lifestyle (Kiehl & Hoffman, 2011; Hare, 1991, 2003). Further, psychopaths are often associated with reactive anger and impulsive violence. Although the PCL-R is considered the "gold standard" in forensic assessment for psychopathy, recent studies have indicated that the reliability may be lower for cases assessed in a clinical or legal setting compared to a research scenario (Edens et al., 2015). To avoid the standard threshold score of the PCL-R as the measure of risk, Edens (2006) suggests the use of a confidence interval to allow for a degree of error, as well as a full understanding of the original utility. Limitations of the PCL-R should be considered when these assessment results are utilized in legal settings.

4.4 Psychopathic Traits in Female Offenders

Most of the literature surrounding psychopathy focuses on males with psychopathic personalities and male offenders, but women with these personality traits are still prevalent within criminal and general populations. In women with psychopathic traits, research has demonstrated some differences in presentation compared to males. Eisenbarth (2014) found that women with psychopathic traits had lower inhibitory deficits but less aggressive behavior. Additionally, highly psychopathic women from the general population demonstrated a stronger correlation between psychopathic traits and self-perception of power and demonstrated more use of manipulation in negotiation situations (Eisenbarth, 2014). Pechorro et al. (2017) found through their research on delinquent girls with psychopathic traits that girls were less likely than boys to be callous and unemotional, possibly because emotional expression and connection to others is more pertinent for women in our society. Understanding these gender differences is valuable when examining and working with women who demonstrate psychopathic personalities. Although they may not demonstrate aggressive or violent behaviors, manipulation may be more prevalent in female offenders with psychopathic traits.

4.5 Psychopathy and the Law

Although there is debate regarding criminality as a key aspect of psychopathy, there is overwhelming evidence (Kiehl & Hoffman, 2011) that individuals with psychopathic traits disproportionately impact the criminal justice system. The common misconception that psychopathic criminals are most often infamous serial killers does not negate the fact that criminals with psychopathic traits are common within the justice system and can be found committing versatile crimes. Interestingly, these numbers may be higher because a psychopath is often deceptive by nature, allowing them to better hide from detection.

Within the law, the psychopathic personality has a complex history. To avoid the use of psychopathy as a potentially excusing mental disorder, the law does not recognize psychopathy as a mental illness and holds individuals with psychopathic personalities responsible for their actions. In 1953, the American Law Institute adopted what has become known as the caveat paragraph in its definition of insanity, excluding some characteristics of psychopathy: "The terms 'mental disease or defect' do not include an abnormality manifested only by repeated criminal or otherwise antisocial conduct" (Kiehl & Hoffman, 2011, p. 9). In 1984, this caveat paragraph was removed from the non-Model Penal Code definition of insanity, but no federal cases since 1984 have utilized psychopathy as a qualifying mental disease (Kiehl & Hoffman, 2011). The presence of psychopathic traits in an individual may blur the lines of responsibility in the eyes of the law. Fine and Kennett (2004) stated that based on Australian law, psychopathic individuals are significantly impaired in moral understanding and do not appear to know why moral transgressions are wrong in the full sense required by the law. However, they argue that detention on the grounds of self-defense, due to severe and continued threat posed by the psychopathic criminal, is appropriate in the case of the psychopathic criminal (Fine & Kennett, 2004).

There are some areas within the law where the concept of psychopathy is utilized, as psychopaths have been found to disproportionately commit certain crimes. Habitual criminal laws, indeterminate sentencing for sex offenders, registration of sex offenders, and special laws on violent sexual predators utilize psychopathy as an indicator of recidivism and violence. Psychopathy is occasionally used to determine dangerousness or risk, ultimately resulting in civil commitment. For example, in the case of sexual psychopaths, individuals can be civilly committed and held for longer than their original sentence when they are deemed "sexual psychopaths." Especially in this case, "psychopath" is synonymous to dangerous, untreatable, and likely to offend again. The American Psychiatric Association opposes these laws and urges the courts to resist the temptation to utilize psychopathy or personality disorders as a direct indicator of violence and recidivism (Fitch, 2000). Gonzalez-Tapia et al. (2017) discuss alternative treatments for psychopaths and the implications of psychopathy within the law. Because of unanswered questions regarding the etiology of psychopathy and inconsistency in the literature, these authors stress there is not a strong scientific bases for reconsidering the current legal treatment of individuals with psychopathic traits. Individuals with psychopathic personalities found within the criminal justice system pose a complex problem, but it is essential to understand and recognize the impact.

4.6   The Criminal Psychopath: What Law Enforcement Needs to Know

For those engaged in law enforcement, it is important to understand criminals with psychopathic traits and skills that can be utilized to effectively manage them. An individual with psychopathic traits may exhibit distinctive behaviors, perceive victims differently, and respond uniquely to interrogation and persecution. In fact, when examining a group of dangerous and severe personalities within a correctional setting, the group had higher psychopathy scores, significantly more convictions before the age of 18 years, greater severity of institutional violence, and more prior crimes of sexual violence compared to the general population (Howard et al., 2012). For the safety of society, as well as law enforcement themselves, recognizing and learning how to effectively identify and manage individuals with this type of personality is critical.

4.6.1   Victimization

Assessing victim vulnerability and victimization is important for law enforcement when preparing for interacting with and interviewing victims of a crime. Wheeler et al. (2009) utilized the Self-Report Psychopathy Scale: Version III (SRP-III) to examine psychopathic traits and perceptions of victim vulnerability. Participants provided a vulnerability estimate for each target while watching short clips of individuals walking. Higher SRP-III scores were associated with greater accuracy in assessing targets' vulnerability to victimization, in other words, victim and nonvictim status (Wheeler et al., 2009). This accuracy was especially significant for those with high Factor 1 (i.e., interpersonal traits) scores, which are related to the ability to read cues of vulnerability in others. Although individuals scoring higher on psychopathic traits were better able to determine who would be a good victim, when prompted they were not able to identify specific cues that indicated vulnerability (Wheeler et al., 2009). This suggests that an individual with psychopathic traits' ability to identify vulnerable victims may not be a conscious decision. Following the choice of a victim, individuals with psychopathic personalities may demonstrate specific forms of abuse and exploitation. Humeny et al. (2020) studied the survivors of psychopathic abusers and assessed their experiences and the psychopathic traits exhibited by their abusers. Abusers with psychopathic traits were associated with the perpetration of domestic abuse that was frequent, versatile, and physically harmful (Humeny et al., 2020). Affective traits were predictive of long-term and versatile abuse, while antisocial traits of psychopathy were associated with the degree of physical injury (Humeny et al., 2020). From the perspective of the survivors of psychopaths, the callousness, unemotionality, and predatory nature provided their abusers with the ability to maintain and escalate the abusive relationship.

4.6.2   Interviewing and Interrogating Individuals with Psychopathic Traits

For law enforcement, effective interrogation techniques are essential when apprehending those who commit crimes. An individual's personality can influence their levels of compliance and the likelihood of a confession. In a study by Larmour et al. (2015), the big five personality traits were the strongest predictors of interrogative compliance (Larmour et al., 2015). Even in an individual not necessarily exhibiting psychopathic traits, understanding personality differences is a tool that law enforcement can use to improve interrogative compliance in an offender. In examining psychopathy exclusively, Larmour et al. (2015) found that the lifestyle facet (e.g., impulsivity, poor behavior control) of psychopathy provided a significant predictor of interrogative compliance. After controlling for the big five personality factors, psychopathy accounted for a small percentage of interrogative compliance, suggesting that taking personality into account is important for law enforcement during an interrogation (Larmour et al., 2015).

Many law enforcement agencies in the United States currently utilize the Reid Technique as a method of interrogating subjects, but these techniques may be less effective when interviewing a psychopathic personality. These traditional techniques could be modified to better address the behavioral and affective differences in an individual with psychopathic traits. These modifications include: *avoiding confrontation, focusing on the collection of inconsistent and implausible facts from the suspect, avoiding threats and mind games, not attempting to appeal to the sympathy, remorse, or regret of the suspect, considering safety issues, and maintaining awareness that strategies should not be altered because of any emotions the suspect displays* (Perri & Lichtenwald, 2008).

A common conception of psychopaths is that they are more likely to participate in lying and malingering when confronted by law enforcement. Malingering includes behaviors like exaggerating an illness to escape duty or work. Because individuals with psychopathic traits may attempt to manipulate others, they may be more likely to use malingering to avoid punishment. But is this the case? The evidence is equivocal. Kucharski et al. (2006) classified a sample of criminal defendants as high, moderate, or low in psychopathy based on PCL-R scores and compared their scores on the MMPI-2, PAI, and SIRS. These assessments are commonly used to detect malingering in offenders. The high psychopathy group scored significantly higher on the tests typically used to detect malingering and that specifically factor 1 of the PCL-R significantly discriminated malingerers from non-malingerers (Kucharski et al., 2006). These results seem to provide evidence that individuals with more psychopathic traits are more likely to malinger; however, further analysis showed that psychopathy ratings had poor sensitivity and specificity in the detection of malingering and that a high percentage of severe psychopaths did not attempt to fake a mental illness (Kucharski et al., 2006). Other researchers found similar patterns, with little relationship between malingering indicators and the Psychopathic Personality Inventory (Poythress et al., 2001). Therefore, psychopathy may not serve as a clinically useful indicator of malingering (Kucharski et al., 2006; Poythress et al., 2001).

4.7 Psychopathic Traits in a Correctional Setting

Within a correctional setting, individuals with psychopathic personalities may exhibit distinctive behaviors that set them apart from their fellow prisoners. Several studies have examined these differences. Utilizing the PCL-R and a behavioral checklist completed by correctional officers, Hobson et al. (2000) found an association with high PCL-R scores and problematic behaviors within prison therapeutic communities. Compared to general inmates, psychopathy was significantly associated with a lower level of involvement in activities such as education, charity work, and wing socials (Hobson et al., 2000). Specifically, when glibness, superficial charm, and a grandiose sense of self-worth were present in individual, these traits were highly correlated with negative behaviors (e.g., "tells lies," "manipulates others") within therapy groups and in the respective wings of the prison. Factor 1 items were associated with negative behavior in the first 6 months of residence (Hobson et al., 2000), as well as less anxious and avoidant traits (Howard et al., 2012), according to the correctional officers working closely with the inmates. Alternatively, Guy et al. (2005) found that Factor 2 items were associated with misconduct in an institutional setting compared to Factor 1 and cautions the use of the PCL-R for forensic decision-making.

Some behaviors exhibited by psychopathic personalities within an institution are not simply disruptive, but also dangerous. Incidents of interpersonal physical aggression were observed for 39% of the dangerous and severe personality disorder sample over an average 1.5-year period following admission (Langton et al., 2011a, b). Dangerous and severe personality disorders in this context included histrionic personality disorder, borderline personality disorder, and antisocial personality disorder. Antisocial personality disorder (assessed utilizing the PCL-R) predicted repetitive incidents of interpersonal physical aggression (Langton et al., 2011a, b). Not only do individuals with psychopathic personalities display interpersonal aggression in a correctional setting, but they may also engage in self-harm behaviors. In fact, a PCL-R total rating of over 30 identified offenders who harmed themselves (Young et al., 2006). Alarmingly, those who harmed themselves were approximately eight times more likely to harm treatment staff (Young et al., 2006).

Due to the foregoing equivocal findings, additional measures may be taken within a correctional facility. Utilizing behavioral checklists may be a useful way to target criminogenic need and identify individuals who may be exhibiting more problem behaviors than others. These checklists may include behaviors that are associated with poor adjustment to a prison environment, as well as psychopathic traits (Hobson et al., 2000). Additionally, instructing staff to identify the types of behaviors shown by psychopaths may be beneficial in managing individuals who demonstrate these personality traits (Hobson et al., 2000). Supplementary training for staff in groupwork skills would also be valuable in preventing psychopaths from disrupting therapy groups (Hobson et al., 2000). These skills might incorporate understanding a group dynamic, conducting a screening for potential group members based on personality traits, and setting realistic expectations for group members.

4.8 Lawyers and Judges

Within the criminal justice system, judges, and lawyers have their own experiences and considerations when working with the psychopathic personality. While judges may encounter individuals with psychopathic traits in their courtroom, attorneys may interact with them as clients or adversaries.

In a psychological evaluation often utilized in court proceedings, a diagnostic label of "psychopath" is not common. Clinicians typically use the Diagnostic and Statistical Manual of Mental Disorders (DSM-5) as a diagnostic tool. In the DSM-5, a diagnostic label of antisocial personality disorder is the only officially diagnosis available for clinicians to specify a psychopathic personality. Not all individuals diagnosed with antisocial personality disorder meet criteria for a label of "psychopath" utilizing the gold standard in psychopathy assessment, the PCL-R. Clinicians utilize antisocial personality disorder liberally among the inmates they diagnose and may look for characteristics more closely associated with the concept of psychopathy (Stevens, 1994). Some clinicians suggest a measure of caution when utilizing PCL-R-based testimony in an adversarial context. Research has demonstrated that experts tended to show partisan allegiance in the way they score the PCL-R (Lloyd et al., 2010).

Edens (2001) provides two case examples that demonstrate the use (or possibly misuse) of the PCL-R in a legal setting. In the first case, PCL-R results were introduced as an *aggravating factor*, or a factor that increases the culpability of a criminal act, in the penalty phase of a capital murder case (Edens, 2001). Alternatively, in the second case, the PCL-R was utilized to *support* expert testimony that a defendant was not likely to be sex offender (Edens, 2001). These cases demonstrate the inconsistency in the use of the PCL-R as evidence of violence potential. Edens (2001) suggests that the presence and absence of psychopathic traits can be misleading as it relates to violence potential, which often depends on the specific context of the case. Examiners should be aware of the settings, circumstances, and populations in which the instrument is appropriate for use, as well as the existing literature on which conclusions are based (Edens, 2001).

4.8.1   Ted Bundy (Rule, 2008)

Ted Bundy was a notorious serial killer executed in 1989 following his conviction for multiple counts of first-degree murder. Bundy admitted to the murder of over 30 young women, as well as assault, kidnapping, and rape. Bundy is widely considered a prolific psychopath, as demonstrated by his gruesome crimes, lack of empathy, callous nature, and infamous charm. In his college years, Bundy studied psychology and later attended law school for some time during his murders. Once Bundy was arrested, he demonstrated notable behaviors that distinguished him from the usual criminal defendant. During his multiple trials, Bundy preferred to act as his own attorney, refusing the advice of his court appointed lawyers and claiming their incompetence regarding his case. Additionally, Bundy successfully escaped custody twice before his final arrest, utilizing manipulation and meticulous planning. Ted Bundy represents not only an extremely violent predator but also a master manipulator who used his egotistical charm to commit deadly crimes and evade capture.

4.8.2 Perceptions of the Justice System

Personality is important in the formation of perceptions of procedural justice, specifically psychopathy. Individuals with psychopathic traits experience a higher rate of encounters with the police and criminal justice system and may perceive these interactions differently than the general population. Psychopathic individuals hold lower perceptions of procedural justice but experience greater increases in their perceptions after involuntary contacts with legal authorities (Augustyn & Ray, 2016). Higher psychopathic traits on the impulsive-irresponsible dimension are specifically associated with these increases, and those with these traits experience a significant increase in perceptions of procedural justice after involuntary encounters with police (Augustyn & Ray, 2016).

4.8.3 Stigma and Labeling

The perception of psychopathic personalities within the courtroom is an important consideration for lawyers and judges. Lawyers specifically should be aware of the negative perceptions of their clients by the jury and understand how these perceptions can affect the outcome of a trial. Research has demonstrated that PCL-R scores are related to trial outcome (Lloyd et al., 2010). Specifically, the label of "psychopath" can have negative connotations that have the power to influence the jury. The idea of consequential validity is an important consideration when labeling a client a psychopath. When examining juror's perceptions of psychopathy, it was found that participant ratings of psychopathy pertaining to the defendant were strongly associated with ratings on measures of his perceived boldness, intelligence, violence potential, and perceptions that he was "evil" (Edens et al., 2013). Additionally, Guy and Edens (2006) found gender differences in the impact of expert testimony regarding psychopathy. Men were less likely than women to support civil commitment when the defendant was described as a "psychopath" (Guy & Edens, 2006). The idea that a defendant is "psychopathic," a word often associate with the loaded term "evil," could greatly contribute to a conviction by the jury.

In the context of juvenile justice, these preemptive labels and the criteria that contributes to these labels can be even more influential. A study examining the effects of these labels on judge's decisions found that the criteria underlying labels of "psychopath" or "conduct disorder" were more influential in juvenile justice contexts than the labels themselves. A history of antisocial behavior was associated with negative effects, while no negative effects were associated with a label of conduct disorder or psychopathy (Murrie et al., 2007). In studies examining jury decisions, a diagnosis of conduct disorder with limited prosocial emotions (a common indicator of future psychopathy) created significant differences in jury decisions. Juveniles with a diagnosis of conduct disorder or limited prosocial emotions were perceived as less amenable to treatment and more dangerous, receiving a more restrictive sentence (Prasad & Kimonis, 2018). Consistent with the findings associated with judges' decisions, participants recommended less restrictive sentences for youth with a diagnosis compared to juveniles showing symptoms but with no diagnostic label (Prasad & Kimonis, 2018). A diagnostic label may illicit sympathy from judges and juries counter to outright behavioral problems. Future researchers may explore the influences of an official diagnosis and how other factors like race may affect the outcomes for juvenile offenders, as these are important considerations for legal decisions. Prasad and Kimonis (2018) suggest the use of comprehensive guidelines for mental health evidence in legal settings to ensure informed decisions that can have significant effects on the lives of young offenders.

4.9   Etiology and Treatment Considerations

Recent research has examined biological aspects of psychopathy. Although genetic and biological mechanisms have been associated with the formation of a psychopathic personality, the law continues to assess psychopaths from a behavioral angle, rather than biological findings (Palermo, 2011). Lawyers and judges may consider the biological bases when making decisions for a defendant. In fact, evidence presented at sentencing in support of a biomechanical cause of the convict's psychopathy significantly reduced the extent to which psychopathy was rated as aggravating and significantly reduced sentencing (Aspinwall et al., 2012). A large consideration in a court proceeding involves the responsibility of the defendant and motivation for their crime. Biological explanations of behavior figure into theories of culpability and punishment (Aspinwall et al., 2012). It is important for the law to further clarify the concept of psychopathy, differentiation between types of psychopaths, and the potential neurobiological correlates (Gonzalez-Tapia et al., 2017).

Individuals with psychopathic traits are widely believed to be resistant to treatment. Research surrounding treatment has not demonstrated much improvement of psychopathic behaviors, possibly due to the lack of motivation by individuals with psychopathic traits to change (Kiehl & Hoffman, 2011). Although promising treatment options for psychopathic traits in juvenile offenders exist (Kiehl & Hoffman, 2011) and the stability of psychopathic traits in children varies (Edens, 2006), there remains little optimism in the treatment of adults, especially within a correctional setting. Clinicians can be influenced by these findings, and psychopathy diagnoses are associated with experts' ratings of treatment amenability, which were related to trial outcome (Lloyd et al., 2010). Some subsets of psychopathic personalities are possibly more amenable to treatment. In fact, Factor 2 psychopaths are more likely to meet criteria for mitigation (Gonzalez-Tapia et al., 2017). These differences indicate that a one-size-fits-all approach to treatment of psychopaths is not optimal. Due to the inconsistency in the literature, there is currently not a strong scientific bases for reconsidering the current legal treatment of psychopaths (Gonzalez-Tapia et al., 2017).

4.10 Psychopathic Traits in Forensic Professionals

4.10.1 Psychopathic Traits in Law Enforcement Professionals

As in all professions, psychopathic traits may be found within individuals serving as law enforcement professionals. Behavioral problems within the police force may signal the existence of an individual with psychopathic personality traits exhibiting risky and violent behavior (Falkenbach et al., 2017, 2018a, b). These traits may lead to misconduct as seen in other examples of successful psychopaths throughout this brief, but may also serve as adaptive characteristics in some first responders (Falkenbach et al., 2018a, b; Lilienfeld et al., 2014; Mullins-Sweatt et al., 2010; Patton et al., 2018).

When examining an urban police sample, some psychopathic traits were identified. Individuals with psychopathic traits were categorized into primary and secondary groups (Falkenbach et al., 2018a, b). The primary group exhibited many of the adaptive traits considered advantageous to police work. These individuals engaged in prosocial behavior inherent in the law enforcement profession and demonstrated fearless dominance (Falkenbach et al., 2018a, b). For those who choose a career in law enforcement, traits like physical risk-taking and emotional distance may be critical for a line of work full of extreme daily physical and emotional stressors (Lilienfeld et al., 2014; Patton et al., 2018). Characteristics of a "successful" psychopath (Mullins-Sweatt et al., 2010) may serve as protective factors from the high-stress environment police officers experience.

In contrast, police officers with secondary psychopathic traits displayed higher levels of aggression and impulsivity and may be more susceptible to "problems" on the job (e.g., police misconduct, aggression) (Falkenbach et al., 2018a, b). Although this study provides preliminary evidence of psychopathic traits contributing to misconduct, there is insufficient research to accurately provide the exact prevalence of these traits within the field of first responders or any causal relationship between these traits and police misconduct. Additionally, police recruits reported higher fearless dominance and coldheartedness scores, while also exhibiting lower self-centered scores (Falkenbach et al., 2018a). Throughout the police recruitment process, safeguards may be in place to identify any individuals who may exhibit characteristics that pose a danger to the community. Psychological testing and background checks (Bannish & Ruiz, 2003) work to filter out applicants who demonstrate psychopathic traits. Although the system is not perfect, police officers who exhibit psychopathic traits may often be terminated from the police forced based on these assessments (Bannish & Ruiz, 2003) or their own poor performance (Bartol, 1991).

Additionally, psychopathic traits may be found within other forensic settings. Quintero et al. (2018) examined the role of empathy and facial emotion recognition abilities of personnel employed at correctional facilities in Mexico. Their results indicated that administrative officers displayed more empathy than security guards, with women exhibiting more empathy than men in general (Quintero et al., 2018).

Empathy and emotion recognition are characteristics that could have implications and effects on the conflicts and social interactions within the correctional setting. Specific training in these areas could have benefits for those working in criminological contexts. Again, results of this study may contribute to our understanding of psychopathic traits within those who enforce the law but is not comprehensive nor definitive.

4.10.2 Police Officers with Psychopathic Traits: Two Case Studies

Through case studies, Falkenbach et al. (2017) demonstrated how psychopathic traits in two urban police officers resulted in divergent outcomes. It is important to note that case studies, on any population in any context, cannot be generalized to the general population. Falkenbach and her colleagues (2017) observed that while the two officers scored high on Factor 1 psychopathic traits (fearless dominance and coldheartedness), they differed on their Factor 2 (self-centered impulsivity) scores and, ultimately, personal and professional outcomes. The officer with low scores on Factor 2 demonstrated an absence of arrest history or discipline resulting from professional misconduct and was likely to obtain promotions throughout his career. However, the officer with high scores on Factor 2 never received a promotion and faced minor disciplinary actions. Additionally, he also had a legal history (e.g., shoplifting) and personal history of socially aversive behaviors (e.g., physical aggression, defiance, manipulation). In this limited snapshot of psychopathic traits in police officers, it is observed that psychopathic traits in police officers may contribute to varying outcomes.

4.10.3 Psychopathic Traits in Lawyers

Lawyers and law students also may exhibit psychopathic traits within their workplace. In lists of occupations where psychopathy is found to be more prevalent, lawyers rank number two (Dutton, 2012). Although no empirical research explicitly examines psychopathy specifically in lawyers, a 2012 JD Candidate Kevin B. Riech wrote a student article addressing the incidence of psychopaths in the legal profession. Riech (2015) described how the series of traits found in psychopathic personalities may exist within lawyers and law students. Interpersonal factors of psychopathy are displayed in habitual dishonesty and "pathological lying traits" potentially found in lawyers whose careers are primarily fueled by money. The affective traits of lack of guilt, callousness, and lack of empathy are also demonstrated by "professional stoicism" sometimes necessary for lawyers. Lifestyle traits characterized by impulsivity are revealed through a strong need for stimulation and a high instance of drug and alcohol abuse. Finally, the antisocial factor of psychopathy related to behavioral issues and criminal tendencies may be identified in some lawyers through their social alienation and isolation. Although Riech's article is based on personal experience and the occasional statistic, his ideas establish a pattern of psychopathic traits that may exist within the legal profession.

4.11 Summary

Learning how to identify individuals with psychopathic traits, the effects they have within this system, and how to work with them effectively is crucial for those working in forensic careers. Psychopaths are 20–25 times more likely than non-psychopaths to be in prison, four to eight times more likely to violently recidivate compared to non-psychopaths, and are resistant to most forms of treatment available within the criminal justice system (Kiehl & Hoffman, 2011). Due to their high prevalence in the criminal justice system, it is likely that law enforcement, lawyers, and judges will encounter these individuals with psychopathic traits. Legally, to avoid the use of psychopathy as a potentially excusing mental disorder, psychopathic traits are not recognized as a mental illness and holds individuals with psychopathic personalities responsible for their actions. However, psychopathic traits and psychopathy assessments are occasionally used to evaluate for future risk, even though the American Psychiatric Association opposes this usage (Fitch, 2000).

An individual with psychopathic traits may exhibit distinctive behaviors, perceive victims differently, and respond uniquely to interrogation and persecution. Within a correctional facility, behaviors of those individuals with psychopathic traits may be unique as well. Lower level of involvement in activities, disruptive behaviors (Hobson et al., 2000), self-harm behaviors (Young et al., 2006), and physical aggression (Langton et al., 2011a, b) may be demonstrated by individuals with psychopathic traits. Specific training and skills may be beneficial for law enforcement and those working within a correctional facility to promote the effective management of these individuals. For lawyers and judges, it is important to understand psychopathic traits and the role they play in the law. The PCL-R is often used (and possibly misused) in a court setting, contributing at times to dangerous assumptions and labeling of offenders that may not accurately reflect their individual responsibility, treatment amenability, or risk of violence.

Additionally, psychopathic traits may be found within those working in a forensic field, including law enforcement and lawyers. Traits like fearless dominance, impulsivity (Falkenbach et al., 2017), and a lack of empathy (Quintero et al., 2018) may be present in law enforcement and correctional officers, leading to possible professional misconduct. Alternatively, these traits may be advantageous in these careers, providing protective factors against ongoing job-related stressors (Falkenbach et al., 2018a, b; Lilienfeld et al., 2014; Mullins-Sweatt et al., 2010; Patton et al., 2018). Riech (2015) also described how the series of traits found in psychopathic personalities may be found within lawyers and law students.

Evaluating for these traits and developing preventative training may be necessary to protect the community as well as other professionals that may encounter these coworkers.

Learning how to identify individuals with psychopathic traits, the effects they have within this system, and how to work with them effectively is crucial for those working in forensic careers. As those in forensic careers are likely to encounter psychopaths as clients, and possibly even coworkers, psychopathy is an important construct to consider.

References

Aspinwall, L. G., Brown, T. R., & Tabery, J. (2012). The double-edged sword: Does biomechanism increase or decrease judges' sentencing of psychopaths? *Science, 337*(6096), 846–849. https://doi.org/10.1126/science.1219569

Augustyn, M. B., & Ray, J. V. (2016). Psychopathy and perceptions of procedural justice. *Journal of Criminal Justice, 46*, 170–183. https://doi.org/10.1016/j.jcrimjus.2016.05.007

Bannish, H., & Ruiz, J. (2003). The antisocial police personality: A view from the inside. *International Journal of Public Administration, 26*(7), 831–881. https://doi.org/10.1081/PAD-120019322

Bartol, C. R. (1991). Predictive validation of the MMPI for small-town police officers who fail. *Professional Psychology: Research and Practice, 22*(2), 127–132. https://doi.org/10.1037/0735-7028.22.2.127

Dutton, K. (2012). *The wisdom of psychopaths: What saints, spies, and serial killers can teach us about success.* Scientific American/Farrar, Straus and Giroux.

Edens, J. F., & Link to external site, this link will open in a new window. (2001). Misuses of the hare psychopathy checklist-revised in court: Two case examples. *Journal of Interpersonal Violence, 16*(10), 1082–1093. https://doi.org/10.1177/088626001016010007

Edens, J. F. (2006). Unresolved controversies concerning psychopathy: Implications for clinical and forensic decision making. *Professional Psychology: Research and Practice; Washington, 37*(1), 59–65. https://doi.org/10.1037/0735-7028.37.1.59

Edens, J. F., Clark, J., Smith, S. T., Cox, J., & Kelley, S. E. (2013). Bold, smart, dangerous and evil: Perceived correlates of core psychopathic traits among jury panel members. *Personality and Mental Health, 7*(2), 143–153. https://doi.org/10.1002/pmh.1221

Edens, J. F., Cox, J., Smith, S. T., DeMatteo, D., & Sörman, K. (2015). How reliable are psychopathy checklist-revised scores in Canadian criminal trials? A case law review. *Psychological Assessment Arlington, 27*(2), 447.

Eisenbarth, H. (2014). Psychopathic personality in women. Diagnostics and experimental findings in the forensic setting and the business world. *Der Nervenarzt, 85*(3), 290, 292–294, 296–297. https://doi.org/10.1007/s00115-013-3902-9

Falkenbach, D. M., Balash, J., Tsoukalas, M., Stern, S., & Lilienfeld, S. O. (2018a). From theoretical to empirical: Considering reflections of psychopathy across the thin blue line. *Personality Disorders: Theory, Research, and Treatment, 9*(5), 420–428. https://doi.org/10.1037/per0000270

Falkenbach, D. M., Glackin, E., & McKinley, S. (2018b). Twigs on the same branch? Identifying personality profiles in police officers using psychopathic personality traits. *Journal of Research in Personality, 76*, 102–112. https://doi.org/10.1016/j.jrp.2018.08.002

Falkenbach, D. M., McKinley, S. J., & Roelofs Larson, F. R. (2017). Two sides of the same coin: Psychopathy case studies from an urban police department. *Journal of Forensic Psychology Research and Practice, 17*(5), 338–356. https://doi.org/10.1080/24732850.2017.1378860

Fine, C., & Kennett, J. (2004). Mental impairment, moral understanding and criminal responsibility: Psychopathy and the purposes of punishment. *International Journal of Law and Psychiatry, 27*(5), 425–443. https://doi.org/10.1016/j.ijlp.2004.06.005

Fitch, W. L. (2000). Law and the confinement of psychopaths. *Behavioral Science & Law, 18,* 16.

Gonzalez-Tapia, M. I., Obsuth, I., & Heeds, R. (2017). A new legal treatment for psychopaths? Perplexities for legal thinkers. *International Journal of Law and Psychiatry, 54,* 46–60. https://doi.org/10.1016/j.ijlp.2017.04.004

Guy, L. S., & Edens, J. F. (2006). Gender differences in attitudes toward psychopathic sexual offenders. *Behavioral Sciences & The Law, 24*(1), 65–85. https://doi.org/10.1002/bsl.665

Guy, L. S., Edens, J. F., Anthony, C., & Douglas, K. S. (2005). Does psychopathy predict institutional misconduct among adults? A meta-analytic investigation. *Journal of Consulting and Clinical Psychology, 73*(6), 1056–1064. https://doi.org/10.1037/0022-006X.73.6.1056

Hare, R. D. (1991). *The hare psychopathy checklist – Revised*. Multi- Health Systems.

Hare, R. D. (2003). *Manual for the revised psychopathy checklist* (2nd ed.). Multi-Health Systems.

Hobson, J., Shine, J., & Roberts, R. (2000). How do psychopaths behave in a prison therapeutic community? *Psychology, Crime & Law, 6*(2), 139–154. https://doi.org/10.1080/10683160008410838

Howard, R., Khalifa, N., Duggan, C., & Lumsden, J. (2012). Are patients deemed "dangerous and severely personality disordered" different from other personality disordered patients detained in forensic settings? *Criminal Behaviour and Mental Health: CBMH, 22*(1), 65. https://doi.org/10.1002/cbm.827

Humeny, C., Forth, A., & Logan, J. (2020). Psychopathic traits predict survivors' experiences of domestic abuse. *Personality and Individual Differences, 110497*. https://doi.org/10.1016/j.paid.2020.110497

Kiehl, K. A., & Hoffman, M. B. (2011). The criminal psychopath: History, neuroscience, treatment, and economics. *Jurimetrics, 51,* 355–397.

Kucharski, L. T., Duncan, S., Egan, S. S., & Falkenbach, D. M. (2006). Psychopathy and malingering of psychiatric disorder in criminal defendants. *Behavioral Sciences & the Law, 24*(5), 633–644. https://doi.org/10.1002/bsl.661

Langton, C. M., Hogue, T. E., Daffern, M., Mannion, A., & Howells, K. (2011a). Personality traits as predictors of inpatient aggression in a high-security forensic psychiatric setting: prospective evaluation of the PCL-R and IPDE dimension ratings. *International Journal of Offender Therapy and Comparative Criminology, 55*(3), 392. https://doi.org/10.1177/0306624X10370828

Langton, C. M., Hogue, T. E., Daffern, M., Mannion, A., & Howells, K. (2011b). Personality traits as predictors of inpatient aggression in a high-security forensic psychiatric setting: Prospective evaluation of the PCL-R and IPDE dimension ratings. *International Journal of Offender Therapy and Comparative Criminology, 55*(3), 392. https://doi.org/10.1177/0306624X10370828

Larmour, S. R., Bergstrøm, H., Gillen, T. A., & C., & Forth, A. E. (2015). Behind the confession: Relating false confession, interrogative compliance, personality traits, and psychopathy. *Journal of Police and Criminal Psychology; Hauppauge, 30*(2), 94. https://doi.org/10.1007/s11896-014-9144-3

Lilienfeld, S. O., Latzman, R. D., Watts, A. L., Smith, S. F., & Dutton, K. (2014). Correlates of psychopathic personality traits in everyday life: Results from a large community survey. *Frontiers in Psychology, 5*. https://doi.org/10.3389/fpsyg.2014.00740

Lloyd, C. D., Clark, H. J., & Forth, A. E. (2010). Psychopathy, expert testimony, and indeterminate sentences: Exploring the relationship between psychopathy checklist-revised testimony and trial outcome in Canada. *Legal and Criminological Psychology, 15*(2), 323–339. https://doi.org/10.1348/135532509X468432

Mullins-Sweatt, S. N., Glover, N. G., Derefinko, K. J., Miller, J. D., & Widiger, T. A. (2010). The search for the successful psychopath. *Journal of Research in Personality, 44*(4), 554–558. https://doi.org/10.1016/j.jrp.2010.05.010

Murrie, D. C., Boccaccini, M. T., McCoy, W., & Cornell, D. G. (2007). Diagnostic labeling in juvenile court: How do descriptions of psychopathy and conduct disorder influence judges? *Journal of Clinical Child and Adolescent Psychology, 36*(2), 228–241. https://doi.org/10.1080/15374410701279602

Palermo, G. B. (2011). Psychopathy: Early and recent clinical observations and the law. *International Journal of Offender Therapy and Comparative Criminology, 55*(1), 3–4. https://doi.org/10.1177/0306624X10395365

Patton, C. L., Smith, S. F., & Lilienfeld, S. O. (2018). Psychopathy and heroism in first responders: Traits cut from the same cloth? *Personality Disorders: Theory, Research, and Treatment, 9*(4), 354–368. https://doi.org/10.1037/per0000261

Pechorro, P., Gonçalves, R. A., Andershed, H., & DeLisi, M. (2017). Female psychopathic traits in forensic and school context: Comparing the antisocial process screening device self-report and the Youth Psychopathic Traits Inventory-Short. *Journal of Psychopathology and Behavioral Assessment, 39*(4), 642–656. https://doi.org/10.1007/s10862-017-9605-y

Perri, F. S., & Lichtenwald, T. G. (2008). Exposing fraud-detection homicide. *The Forensic Examiner, 17*(1), 26–33.

Poythress, N. G., Edens, J. F., & Watkins, M. M. (2001). The relationship between psychopathic personality features and malingering symptoms of major mental illness. *Law and Human Behavior, 25*(6), 567–582.

Prasad, A. H., & Kimonis, E. R. (2018). Effects of the "limited prosocial emotions" specifier for conduct disorder on juror perceptions of juvenile offenders. *Criminal Justice and Behavior, 45*(10), 1547–1564. https://doi.org/10.1177/0093854818774381

Quintero, L. A. M., Muñoz-Delgado, J., Sánchez-Ferrer, J. C., Fresán, A., Brüne, M., & Arango de Montis, I. (2018). Facial emotion recognition and empathy in employees at a Juvenile detention center. *International Journal of Offender Therapy and Comparative Criminology, 62*(8), 2430–2446. https://doi.org/10.1177/0306624X17721518

Riech, K. B. (2015). Psycho lawyer, qu'est-ce que c'est: the high incidence of psychopaths in the legal profession and why they thrive. *Law and Psychology Review, 39*, 287–299.

Rule, A. (2008). *The stranger beside me*. Pocket Books.

Stevens, G. F. (1994). Prison clinicians' perceptions of antisocial personality disorder as a formal diagnosis. *Journal of Offender Rehabilitation, 20*(3–4), 159–185. https://doi.org/10.1300/J076v20n03_10

Wheeler, S., Book, A., & Costello, K. (2009). Psychopathic traits and perceptions of victim vulnerability. *Criminal Justice and Behavior, 36*(6), 635–648. https://doi.org/10.1177/0093854809333958

Young, M. H., Justice, J. V., & Erdberg, P. (2006). Risk of harm: Inmates who harm themselves while in prison psychiatric treatment. *Journal of Forensic Sciences, 51*(1), 156–162. https://doi.org/10.1111/j.1556-4029.2005.00023.x

Chapter 5
Education

5.1 Introduction

Psychopathy within education is explored from three different domains: school age youths, college students, and professionals working within an academic setting. Individuals at the college or professional levels share considerable overlap with corporate psychopathy, with some corporate psychopathy research focusing on business students as future leaders (Sekhar et al., 2020) or defining academia as akin to corporate structures (Pheko, 2018). In many ways, those with psychopathic traits in education are considered successful psychopaths. Success has been described in a variety of ways in the literature; however, within education, success is commonly ascribed to those reaching professional achievement (Forster & Lund, 2018; Pheko, 2018) or being admitted to a college level program (e.g., Mullins-Nelson et al., 2006). Importantly, the moniker of success is often delineated by incarceration, as unsuccessful psychopaths are typically found in forensic settings due to their inability to operate within legal boundaries (Skeem et al., 2011). On the other hand, psychopathic traits in children may be differentially expressed based on factors such as childhood abuse (e.g., Kimonis et al., 2012) and parenting style (e.g., Frick & White, 2008). Early intervention is crucial for children who exhibit psychopathic traits, as maladaptive behaviors are more likely to worsen over time (Ribeiro da Silva et al., 2020). However, experts have long debated the mechanisms underlying the development of psychopathy (Salekin & Lynam, 2010). As psychopathic individuals are a heterogeneous population encompassing a variety of behaviors, some scholars have begun conceptualizing psychopathy as more of a continuum rather than a singular category (Sellbom & Drislane, 2020).

5.2   Prevalence

One of the many challenges of determining prevalence of psychopathic traits in educational settings is the lack of epidemiological studies focused on this population. No conclusive evidence was found to determine the specific prevalence of psychopathy within school age children, college students, or college employees. The prevalence of psychopathy in children may be inferred from adult samples, which are estimated at approximately 1% of the general population (Hare, 1998). Large-scale epidemiological studies have estimated the prevalence of antisocial personality disorder (ASPD) at about 1–4% of the general population (Lenzenweger et al., 2007; Trull et al., 2010). However, while ASPD shares some overlap, psychopathy encompasses a more complex array of features.

Many of the studies provided on school age children (e.g., Vaughn et al., 2010; DeLisi et al., 2011; Fanti & Kimonis, 2013) and college students (e.g., Hassall et al., 2015; Litten et al., 2018, 2020) examine psychopathy through the lens of high and low psychopathic traits, rather than through the dichotomy of psychopathic or not. Conceptualizing psychopathy as a constellation of traits (Sellbom & Drislane, 2020) is especially useful for understanding subclinical psychopathy (i.e., individuals that fall below the common threshold for a "psychopath" label) as the presence of psychopathic traits may still contribute to maladaptive interpersonal and behavioral characteristics (e.g., Mouilso & Calhoun, 2013; Hassall et al., 2015; Lee et al., 2020).

5.3   Psychopathy in Children

The use of the term psychopathy as it applies to children is largely debated in the literature. Some argue that children undergo a series of changes to their personality as they develop and that labeling children with psychopathy is both difficult to accurately determine and potentially damaging (Edens & Vincent, 2008). However, personality is generally stable throughout the lifespan of an individual, and normative changes in development do not preclude the presence of personality disorders in children (Lynam et al., 2009). Further, there is evidence for stability of psychopathic traits over the course of longitudinal studies (Frick et al., 2003; Lynam et al., 2009). Psychopathy intervention research highlights the importance of early identification and intervention as a necessity for reducing maladaptive outcomes (Pisano et al., 2017). Several intervention strategies have shown promise for the treatment of callous-unemotional traits and conduct problems. Unfortunately, school faculty are limited in there ability to provide direct intervention. While school personnel may contribute to the behavioral ratings of students to track progress (e.g., Lochman et al., 2015), intervention strategies are typically given outside of a school setting by trained professionals (e.g., clinicians, doctoral students; Wilkinson et al., 2016; Pisano et al., 2017).

5.3.1 Primary Versus Secondary Psychopathy

Much like adults, research regarding children with psychopathic traits points to psychopathy subtypes (e.g., Kimonis et al., 2012; Kahn et al., 2013; Huang et al., 2019), specifically indicating primary and secondary psychopathy presentations within children. Children deemed as having psychopathic traits largely differ regarding early childhood experiences (Kimonis et al., 2012). Theoretically, children with primary psychopathy will typically demonstrate more callous unemotional traits (e.g., lack of empathy, not caring of how their behavior affects others; Karpman, 1941) and fearlessness (Lykken, 1995). Children with primary psychopathy are less emotionally reactive and commonly show affective deficits. On the other hand, emotional problems may be the main indicator of secondary psychopathy, which is thought to develop in response to adverse childhood experiences, such as abuse or trauma (Kimonis et al., 2012).

In this context, emotional problems relate to increased startle responses that may manifest as problems of emotional regulation and reactivity (Kimonis et al., 2017). This could ultimately lead to increases in conduct problems and future criminality. Conduct problems defined by McMahon et al. (2006) include "a broad range of 'acting-out' behaviors, ranging from annoying but relatively minor oppositional behaviors (such as yelling and temper tantrums) to more serious forms of antisocial behavior (including aggression, physical destructiveness, and stealing)" (p. 137). For example, Weiler and Widom (1996) found individuals who have been abused or neglected in childhood had higher PCL-R scores than controls. High PCL-R scores in this sample positively predicted criminal history. However, early childhood victimization itself is not a predictor of criminality when controlling for psychopathy (Weiler & Widom, 1996). Huang et al. (2019) propose that children who fall under the umbrella of psychopathy can be differentiated by their level of anxiety. Children with psychopathic traits were divided into two subgroups, a "primary variant" (i.e., high in callous-unemotional traits and conduct problems) and a "secondary variant" (i.e., high in callous-unemotional traits, conduct problems, and anxiety). Both subgroups of children with psychopathic traits demonstrated more conduct problems than normal or anxious peers. However, the "secondary variant" exhibited the most conduct problems of any group, indicating that anxiety could play an integral role in the occurrence of conduct issues (Huang et al., 2019).

5.3.2 Parenting Can Play a Role

Lilienfeld et al. (2015) propose positive parenting styles may moderate the expression of psychopathy. Positive parenting has the potential to reduce callous-unemotional traits later in life (Frick & White, 2008; Waller et al., 2013). For example, Frick et al. (2003) followed a group 98 school-age students to assess the stability of psychopathic traits across a four-year period. The authors found poor parenting (e.g., inadequate parental monitoring, a lack of consistent discipline) was associated with antisocial behaviors at follow-up. Whereas in cases of reduced callous-unemotional traits, positive parenting (e.g., higher parental involvement and use of positive reinforcement) was found to be a significant factor (Frick et al., 2003). These findings were consistent with the research by Hawes et al. (2011), which revealed a similar relationship between parenting quality and callous-unemotional traits after one year.

5.3.3   Psychopathy in the Classroom

Research in the field predominantly focuses on children who act out through maladaptive means, sometimes resulting in criminality and subsequent incarceration. As such, most research revolves around juveniles within a forensic context. There is little known about how psychopathy manifests in the classroom. However, children who are disruptive or antisocial within educational settings frequently experience other difficulties such as interpersonal problems with peers (e.g., bullying; Walsh et al., 2018), deficits in academic achievement, and an increase in externalizing behaviors (DeLisi et al., 2011).

There are significant comorbidities between attention deficit hyperactivity disorder (ADHD), oppositional defiant disorder (ODD), and conduct disorder (CD; American Psychiatric Association, 2013), which are often associated with externalizing behavioral problems (e.g., bullying; Ghosh & Sinha, 2012). Children with ODD and CD are more likely to exhibit psychopathic traits (e.g., callous unemotional traits, impulsivity) that may persist into adulthood. According to Lynam's (1996) "fledgling psychopaths" theory, children exhibiting conduct problems in combination with hyperactivity, impulsivity, and attention deficits will likely present as having severe CD. These children may carry psychopathic traits into adulthood and are at higher risk of becoming chronic offenders (Lynam, 1996). DeLisi et al. (2011) investigated "fledgling psychopathy" on educational outcomes in a classroom sample of 432 adolescents. The results indicated that individuals from all three ADHD groups (i.e., hyperactive-impulsive, inattentive, and mixed-type hyperactive-impulsive/inattentive) had significantly more callous-unemotional traits when compared with control group peers. Both the inattentive and mixed-type ADHD groups demonstrated poor test performance (e.g., reading comprehension). The mixed-type students presented with comparatively higher psychopathic traits (e.g., callous-unemotional and behavioral problems) than all other groups, coupled with the lowest IQs and testing scores. Students within the hyperactive-impulsive group had higher IQ scores and did not perform poorly on educational measures (DeLisi et al., 2011). Theoretically, poor performance in school and on educational measures may also be linked to the affective deficits in children with callous-unemotional traits (Vaughn et al., 2010; DeLisi et al., 2011). For example, reading tasks could require a certain level of emotional competence that is lacking in children with psychopathic traits (Vaughn et al., 2010). This lack of empathy may extend to facets of school-based behavior such as underperformance due to indifference toward academic achievement (Vaughn et al., 2010, DeLisi et al., 2011).

5.3.4 Bullying

Bullying behavior is an externalizing behavior often seen in children with psychopathic traits and/or conduct disorder. Bullying is characterized as "aggression involving the repeated and systematic abuse of power in a relationship" (Walsh et al., 2018, p.3) and encompasses a range of behaviors such as mocking, name calling, pushing, and hitting (Ragatz et al., 2011). Retrospective studies utilized college samples to identify participation in bullying or being victimized during their adolescent years. These studies found that bullies and those who fell into a mixed category (i.e., being both the victim of bullying, but also participating in bullying others) reported significantly more psychopathic traits than victim and control groups (Ragatz et al., 2011; Walsh et al., 2018). Bullying groups were found to display higher levels of proactive aggression (e.g., associated with more callous traits, planned and done with purpose), whereas the mixed-type group engaged in more reactive aggression (e.g., relates to poor emotional control, impulsivity; Ragatz et al., 2011). Interestingly, the results from Walsh et al. (2018) indicate that compared to controls, both the bully group and victim group were higher on empathy measures that relate to the understanding of others' emotions. Another study found those with callous unemotional traits are more likely to engage in bullying behaviors (Fanti & Kimonis, 2013). One longitudinal study conducted by Fanti and Kimonis (2013) followed a group of 1416 adolescents to determine whether psychopathic traits (e.g., narcissism, impulsivity, callous-unemotional, and conduct problems) could predict bullying or victimization. Their findings suggest narcissism, impulsivity, and callous-unemotional traits all contribute to bullying and are most likely to occur when all three factors are present within an individual. High levels of narcissism were more likely to be present in bullies than bullying victims. In contrast, impulsivity in adolescents predicted later increases in victimization (Fanti & Kimonis, 2013).

5.4 Psychopathy in Higher Education

5.4.1 Academic Majors

College samples are widely utilized in academic research; however, investigations into the effects of psychopathy on college students within an educational setting are less common. Literature regarding psychopathy in corporate leaders (e.g., Babiak et al., 2010; Boddy, 2011) has seemingly inspired researchers to investigate how psychopathy may influence academic pursuits.

Theoretically, individuals with higher levels of psychopathic traits may gravitate to certain fields of study (e.g., business) because of perceived benefit and status (Krick et al., 2016). However, the myth that psychopaths exclusively choose business majors is misguided, as varying degrees of psychopathic traits appear throughout majors (e.g., Wilson & McCarthy, 2011; Krick et al., 2016; Vedel & Thomsen, 2017). Researchers have begun to explore how psychopathic traits may contribute to the selection of academic majors (Wilson & McCarthy, 2011; Hassall et al., 2015; Krick et al., 2016; Vedel & Thomsen, 2017; Litten et al., 2020). Some studies limited the scope of their sample to business and psychology majors (Hassall et al., 2015; Litten et al., 2018; Litten et al., 2020). While other research included an array of fields, such as engineering, sciences, humanities (e.g., Krick et al., 2016), law, and political science majors (e.g., Vedel & Thomsen, 2017). Notably, there appears to be a stark contrast between business majors and those in helping professions, such as psychology. Business students have significantly more psychopathic traits when compared to psychology students (Hassall et al., 2015; Litten et al., 2018; Vedel & Thomsen, 2017; Litten et al., 2020). Hassall et al. (2015) examined psychopathic traits using a four-factor approach (e.g., interpersonal manipulation, callous affect, erratic lifestyle, and antisocial behavior). The results suggest business students tend to be more psychopathic, as they scored higher than psychology students on all four factors. Empathy may be an important component to major selection between business and psychology students, as business students typically score lower on empathy measures (Litten et al., 2018; Litten et al., 2020). However, results from Vedel and Thomsen (2017) suggest these differences in psychopathy are insignificant when comparing business students to political science and law students.

Irrespective of degree choice, men scored higher on psychopathic measures than women (Wilson & McCarthy, 2011; Krick et al., 2016; Vedel & Thomsen, 2017). Additionally, while it may appear psychopathic traits are more concentrated in certain academic disciplines based on proportion of males within a chosen major, psychopathy was still seen in a predominantly female sample of law students (Vedel & Thomsen, 2017). Interestingly, psychopathy was not found to predict the selection of academic major (Vedel & Thomsen, 2017; Litten et al., 2020). While psychopathic traits are present across a variety of majors, research points to a higher concentration of these traits within academic disciplines relating to business (Wilson & McCarthy, 2011; Hassall et al., 2015; Krick et al., 2016; Vedel & Thomsen, 2017; Litten et al., 2020).

5.4.2   Academic and Cheating Behaviors

Hassall and colleagues (2016) identified gender and antisocial behavior as important predictors of academic success. Their findings suggest that men with higher levels of antisocial behavior achieve lower grades than their peers (Hassall et al., 2015). A longitudinal study conducted by Dworkin and Widom (1977) examined life outcomes of individuals classified as having psychopathic deviate profiles in college. Individuals with psychopathic traits were less likely to complete a graduate level degree than those with normal profiles. However, the groups did not differ significantly on schooling beyond college, this may imply higher dropout rates for psychopathic students in graduate school. Their findings indicate that high levels of intelligence do not preclude individuals with psychopathic traits from negative outcomes (Dworkin & Widom, 1977). For instance, poor grades can be indicative of cognitive deficits that may motivate cheating behaviors as a method of compensation (Paulhus & Dubois, 2015).

Academic dishonesty in the form of cheating (e.g., plagiarism, cheating on assignments, cheating on tests) is a concern for academic institutions. Research has demonstrated a connection between cheating (e.g., attitudes and behaviors) and personality features like psychopathic traits (Lee et al., 2020; Williams et al., 2010; Coyne & Thomas, 2008). Williams et al. (2010) conducted research relating to psychopathy and cheating in a sample of 249 undergraduate students. The authors found it prudent to ask students about cheating during their high school years to help control for inaccurate self-reports. Individuals who were high in psychopathic traits admitted to cheating more frequently than their peers. Furthermore, psychopathy was predictive of cheating behaviors over and above the other Dark Triad traits (i.e., Machiavellianism, narcissism; Williams et al., 2010). In a large-scale meta-analytic review by Lee et al. (2020), psychopathy and impulsivity (which is often included as a dimension of psychopathy) were found to be significant predictors of academic dishonesty. Impulsivity is thought to potentially differentiate primary from secondary psychopathy (Ray et al., 2009), as secondary psychopaths typically exhibit more impulsivity associated with maladaptive behaviors such as criminal behavior (Gray et al., 2019). While impulsivity was found to be predictive of academic dishonesty (Lee et al., 2020), the findings from Coyne and Thomas (2008) demonstrated that within their sample, cheating was associated with primary but not secondary psychopathy.

5.4.3 Psychopathic College Students and Aggression

College students with high psychopathic traits are more inclined to engage in aggressive behaviors toward others (Kosson et al., 1997; Mouilso & Calhoun, 2013; Lago-Gonzalez et al., 2021). Students high in psychopathic trait are more likely to use manipulation to endanger and harm the interpersonal relationships of their peers (i.e., relational aggression). Additionally, psychopathy has been found to predict the use of proactive (i.e., intentional and calculated behavior to achieve an objective) and reactive (i.e., rash decisions based on emotional upset) relational aggression (Knight et al., 2018). Aggressive behaviors can also include actual or threaten physical assault. For example, college males with psychopathic traits report engaging in significantly more sexual aggression (Kosson et al., 1997; Mouilso & Calhoun, 2013, see Psychopathic college students and sexual aggression). Lago-Gonzalez and colleagues (2020) investigated psychopathic and borderline traits as they relate to aggression, in a sample of 622 French college students. Students high in psychopathic traits tend to report more aggression toward others (e.g., attempting to cause physical harm to another person, engaging in behaviors to aggravate someone). Individuals that were high on both borderline and psychopathic traits engaged in aggression toward others and the self (e.g., self-injurious behaviors, suicidal attempts; Lago-Gonzalez et al., 2021). However, it is important to note the authors caution the generalizability of these findings to populations outside of France. More research is needed to explore aggression and psychopathy in college samples.

5.4.4 Psychopathic College Students and Sexual Aggression

Within forensic populations there is a long-standing association between psychopathic traits and sexual violence. Alarmingly, college students exhibiting psychopathic traits are more likely than their peers to commit sexual assault (Kosson et al., 1997; Mouilso & Calhoun, 2013). Sexual assault on college campuses is a pervasive problem. According to a national survey of 181,752 students across 33 campuses, the rate of nonconsensual sexual contact was approximately 13%. Sexual victimization was found to disproportionately affect undergraduate women (25.9%) and undergraduates that identified as transgender, nonbinary/genderqueer, gender questioning, or did not list their gender (22.8%; Cantor et al., 2017). Arguably, sexual assault is more common in colleges because of rape culture, which includes the acceptance of rape myths.

There are several definitions of rape myths. For instance, the Rape Myth Acceptance Scale (RMAS) operationalize rape myths as the "prejudicial, stereotyped or false beliefs about rape, rape victims, and rapists" (Burt, 1980 p. 217). Lonsway and Fitzgerald (1994, p. 134) describe rape myths as "attitudes and beliefs that are generally false, but are widely and persistently held, and that serve to deny and justify male sexual aggression against women." In general, the overarching theme of what constitutes rape myths encompasses false beliefs regarding rape that are pervasive and inaccurate (Edwards et al., 2011). Some common examples of rape myths include: (a) women who wear tight or revealing clothing are asking to be raped, (b) women secretly want to be raped, (c) women cannot be raped by their husbands, (d) women like being raped, (e) false rape allegations are a prevalent problem, and (f) women lie about rape (Edwards et al., 2011). They are applied within a society to make sexual aggression seem innocuous (Payne et al., 1994).

Psychopathy is associated with negative attitudes toward rape victims (Watts et al., 2017) and perpetration of sexual assault (Kosson et al., 1997). Generally, college students and alumni are less likely to hold false ideas about rape and tend to be more compassionate to rape victims (Ferro et al., 2008). However, the same trend is not seen among college students with psychopathic traits. Students with psychopathic traits frequently endorse rape myths (Mouilso & Calhoun, 2013; Watts et al.,

2017; Cooke et al., 2020) and have more positive attitudes toward sexual coercion (O'Connell & Marcus, 2016). Furthermore, Watts et al. (2017) found that psychopathic traits, such as disinhibition and meanness, predict rape myth acceptance. However, experiences in childhood and adolescence (e.g., psychological victimization by a caregiver) may indirectly impact rape myth acceptance. Cooke et al. (2020), propose this type of psychological victimization relates to increased psychopathic traits in men (e.g., egocentricity), which in turn is associated with greater acceptance of rape myths.

Importantly, the association between psychopathy and sexual violence is not limited to attitudes alone. A study conducted by Mouilso and Calhoun (2013) investigated the associations among psychopathy and rape myth acceptance on self-reported sexual assault perpetration in a sample of 308 undergraduate males. The authors found that individuals with higher psychopathic traits were more likely to not only accept rape myths but commit acts of sexual aggression (e.g., unwanted sexual contact, rape). This outcome relates to previous research which found psychopathic traits in college males were able to predict self-reports of sexual aggression (e.g., threats and use of force; Kosson et al., 1997).

5.4.5 Psychopathic Leadership in Academic Settings

Within the sometimes-toxic environment of academia, the presence of unscrupulous department heads or abusive faculty can appear pervasive. However, the effects of psychopathy in academia are largely theoretical (Perry, 2015; Forster & Lund, 2018). These studies reference previous research discussing successful psychopathy in the workplace as a template for how psychopathy might impact higher education. Arguably academic leaders with Dark Triad traits (i.e., narcissism, Machiavellianism, and psychopathy) may be able to disrupt collaborative efforts essential to the quality and function of higher education (Perry, 2015). Forster and Lund (2018) describe universities as subject to a diffusion of power that allows more freedom to established faculty (e.g., tenured professors) then would commonly be seen in a corporate structure. Notably, this power may be wielded by faculty to bully others (Forster & Lund, 2018).

Little research has specifically investigated psychopathy in faculty employed within higher education. Pheko (2018) conducted a qualitative study that included four cases of faculty who reported bullying and mobbing during their employment at a university located in Botswana. The four individuals worked within the field of psychology at the time of the alleged incidents. Bullying took the form of a variety of manipulative and deceptive behaviors, ranging from spreading misinformation to fabricating documents. Based on these accounts the author theorized that psychopathic perpetrators of bullying behavior often utilized "rumors and gossip" to humiliate subordinates. The faculty members who were victimized by this behavior believe that bullying behaviors directly impacted their promotional opportunities as well as their employment status (Pheko, 2018).

5.5   Summary

Evidence points to the existence of primary and secondary psychopathy within children exhibiting psychopathic traits (e.g., Kimonis et al., 2012; Kahn et al., 2013; Huang et al., 2019). As secondary psychopathy tends to vary based on emotional dysregulation, potentially developing from adverse childhood experiences (Kimonis et al., 2012), it is often associated with maladaptive outcomes (e.g., criminal behavior; Weiler & Widom,1996). Commonly, callous-unemotional traits are associated with primary psychopathy (Kahn et al., 2013); however, Huang et al. (2019) present evidence that secondary psychopathy in children is determined by anxiety, and callous-unemotional traits are present in both groups. Research regarding "fledgling psychopathy" in the classroom has been associated with inattention, callous-unemotional traits, increased behavioral problems, and poor performance on reading tasks (DeLisi et al., 2011). Behavioral problems have been linked to psychopathic traits and may manifest as aggression such as bullying (e.g., Ragatz et al., 2011).

Literature regarding successful psychopathy as it pertains to the corporate world has been influential to research efforts geared toward psychopathy in academic settings (e.g., Wilson & McCarthy, 2011; Hassall et al., 2015; Pheko, 2018). Theoretical exploration of psychopathy in higher educational leadership has identified the potential for psychopathic traits to negatively impact collaborative efforts within their departments (Perry, 2015). Additionally, researchers have begun to explore the effects of psychopathic traits in areas such as the selection of majors, academic dishonesty, and aggression. Research has consistently found individuals with psychopathic traits tend to choose business-related fields of study (e.g., Wilson & McCarthy, 2011; Hassall et al., 2015; Krick et al., 2016). While psychopathy does not predict academic major choice (e.g., Vedel & Thomsen, 2017), differences in empathy have been identified as a key factor for selection (Litten et al., 2018; Litten et al., 2020). Psychopathic traits are associated with maladaptive behaviors and choices in college settings. College students scoring higher in psychopathy are more likely to cheat (e.g., Williams et al., 2010), as well as exhibit aggressive and violent behaviors toward peers (e.g., Kosson et al., 1997; Mouilso & Calhoun, 2013).

This review aimed to provide a brief overview of the literature focused on psychopathy in educational settings. As psychopathic traits encompass a range of maladaptive behaviors and outcomes, individuals working within this field may benefit from identifying common behaviors and traits presented. However, research in this area is limited. Further investigation is needed to explore the prevalence and role of psychopathy within all facets of education.

References

American Psychiatric Association. (2013). Anxiety disorders. In *Diagnostic and statistical manual of mental disorders* (5th ed.). https://doi.org/10.1176/appi.books.9780890425596.dsm05

Babiak, P., Neumann, C. S., & Hare, R. D. (2010). Corporate psychopathy: Talking the walk. *Behavioral Sciences & the Law*, n/a–n/a. https://doi.org/10.1002/bsl.925

Boddy, C. R. (2011). Corporate psychopaths, bullying and unfair supervision in the workplace. *Journal of Business Ethics, 100*(3), 367–379. https://doi.org/10.1007/s10551-010-0689-5

Burt, M. R. (1980). Cultural myths and supports for rape. *Journal of Personality and Social Psychology, 38*(2), 217–230. https://doi.org/10.1037/0022-3514.38.2.217

Cantor, D., Fisher, B., Chibnall, S., Harps, S., Townsend, R., Thomas, G., Lee, H., Kranz, V., Herbison, R., & Madden, K. (2017). *Report on the AAU Campus Climate Survey on Sexual Assault and Misconduct.* 433.

Cooke, E. M., Lewis, R. H., Hayes, B. E., Bouffard, L. A., Boisvert, D. L., Wells, J., Kavish, N., Woeckener, M., & Armstrong, T. A. (2020). Examining the relationship between victimization, psychopathy, and the acceptance of rape myths. *Journal of Interpersonal Violence, 088626052096666.* https://doi.org/10.1177/0886260520966669

Coyne, S. M., & Thomas, T. J. (2008). Psychopathy, aggression, and cheating behavior: A test of the cheater–hawk hypothesis. *Personality and Individual Differences, 44*(5), 1105–1115. https://doi.org/10.1016/j.paid.2007.11.002

DeLisi, M., Vaughn, M., Beaver, K. M., Wexler, J., Barth, A. E., & Fletcher, J. M. (2011). Fledgling psychopathy in the classroom: ADHD subtypes, psychopathy, and reading comprehension in a community sample of adolescents. *Youth Violence and Juvenile Justice, 9*(1), 43–58. https://doi.org/10.1177/1541204010371932

Dworkin, R. H., & Widom, C. S. (1977). Undergraduate MMPI Profiles and the Longitudinal Prediction of Adult Social Outcome, p. 5.

Edens, J. F., & Vincent, G. M. (2008). Juvenile psychopathy: A clinical construct in need of restraint? *Journal of Forensic Psychology Practice, 8*(2), 186–197. https://doi.org/10.1080/15228930801964042

Edwards, K. M., Turchik, J. A., Dardis, C. M., Reynolds, N., & Gidycz, C. A. (2011). Rape myths: History, individual and institutional-level presence, and implications for change. *Sex Roles: A Journal of Research, 65*(11-12), 761–773. https://doi.org/10.1007/s11199-011-9943-2

Fanti, K. A., & Kimonis, E. R. (2013). Dimensions of juvenile psychopathy distinguish "bullies," "bully-victims," and "victims". *Psychology of Violence, 3*(4), 396–409. https://doi.org/10.1037/a0033951

Ferro, C., Cermele, J., & Saltzman, A. (2008). Current perceptions of marital rape: Somegood and not-so-good news. *Journal of Interpersonal Violence, 23*(6), 764–779. https://doi.org/10.1177/0886260507313947

Forster, N., & Lund, D. W. (2018). Identifying and dealing with functional psychopathic behavior in higher education. *Global Business and Organizational Excellence, 38*(1), 22–31. https://doi.org/10.1002/joe.21897

Frick, P. J., & White, S. F. (2008). Research review: The importance of callous-unemotional traits for developmental models of aggressive and antisocial behavior. *Journal of Child Psychology and Psychiatry, 49*(4), 359–375. https://doi.org/10.1111/j.1469-7610.2007.01862.x

Frick, P. J., Cornell, A. H., Barry, C. T., Bodin, S. D., & Dane, H. E. (2003). Callous-unemotional traits and conduct problems in the prediction of conduct problem severity, Aggression, and Self-Report of Delinquency, *14.*

Ghosh, S., & Sinha, M. (2012). ADHD, ODD, and CD: Do they belong to a common psychopathological Spectrum? A case series. *Case reports in psychiatry, 2012, 520689.* https://doi.org/10.1155/2012/520689

Gray, N. S., Weidacker, K., & Snowden, R. J. (2019). Psychopathy and impulsivity: The relationship of psychopathy to different aspects of UPPS-P impulsivity. *Psychiatry Research, 272,* 474–482. https://doi.org/10.1016/j.psychres.2018.12.155

Hare, R. D. (1998). Psychopaths and their nature: Implications for the mental health and criminal justice systems. In T. Millon, E. Simonsen, M. Birket-Smith, & R. D. Davis (Eds.), *Psychopathy: Antisocial, criminal, and violent behavior* (pp. 188–212). The Guilford Press. (This chapter is a revised and updated version of a paper that first appeared in Criminal Justice and Behavior, 1996, 23, pp. 25–54).

Hassall, J., Boduszek, D., & Dhingra, K. (2015). Psychopathic traits of business and psychology students and their relationship to academic success. *Personality and Individual Differences, 82,* 227–231. https://doi.org/10.1016/j.paid.2015.03.017

Hawes, D. J., Dadds, M. R., Frost, A. D. J., & Hasking, P. A. (2011). Do childhood callous-unemotional traits drive change in parenting practices? *Journal of Clinical Child & Adolescent Psychology, 40*(4), 507–518. https://doi.org/10.1080/15374416.2011.581624

Huang, J., Fan, L., Lin, K., & Wang, Y. (2019). Variants of children with psychopathic tendencies in a community sample. *Child Psychiatry & Human Development, 51*(4), 563–571. https://doi.org/10.1007/s10578-019-00939-9

Kahn, R. E., Frick, P. J., Youngstrom, E. A., Youngstrom, J. K., Feeny, N. C., & Findling, R. L. (2013). Distinguishing primary and secondary variants of callous-unemotional traits among adolescents in a clinic-referred sample 14.

Karpman, B. (1941). On the need of separating psychopathy into two distinct clinical types: The symptomatic and the idiopathic. *Journal of Criminal Psychopathology, 3*, 112–137.

Kimonis, E. R., Frick, P. J., Cauffman, E., Goldweber, A., & Skeem, J. (2012). Primary and secondary variants of juvenile psychopathy differ in emotional processing. *Development and Psychopathology, 24*(3), 1091–1103. https://doi.org/10.1017/S0954579412000557

Kimonis, E. R., Fanti, K. A., Goulter, N., & Hall, J. (2017). Affective startle potentiation differentiates primary and secondary variants of juvenile psychopathy. *Development and Psychopathology, 29*(4), 1149–1160. https://doi.org/10.1017/S0954579416001206

Knight, N. M., Dahlen, E. R., Bullock-Yowell, E., & Madson, M. B. (2018). The HEXACO model of personality and dark triad in relational aggression. *Personality and Individual Differences, 122*, 109–114. https://doi.org/10.1016/j.paid.2017.10.016

Kosson, D. S., Kelly, J. C., & White, J. W. (1997). Psychopathy-related traits predict self-reported sexual aggression among college men. *Journal of Interpersonal Violence, 12*(2), 241–254. https://doi.org/10.1177/088626097012002006

Krick, A., Tresp, S., Vatter, M., Ludwig, A., Wihlenda, M., & Rettenberger, M. (2016). The relationships between the dark triad, the moral judgment level, and the students' disciplinary choice: Self-selection, indoctrination, or both? *Journal of Individual Differences, 37*(1), 24–30. https://doi.org/10.1027/1614-0001/a000184

Lago-Gonzalez, L., Bronchain, J., & Chabrol, H. (2021). Psychopathic and borderline traits in a college sample: Personality profiles and relations to self-directed and other-directed aggression. *Personality and Individual Differences, 168*, 110390. https://doi.org/10.1016/j.paid.2020.110390

Lee, S. D., Kuncel, N. R., & Gau, J. (2020). Personality, attitude, and demographic correlates of academic dishonesty: A meta-analysis. *Psychological Bulletin, 146*(11), 1042–1058. https://doi.org/10.1037/bul0000300

Lenzenweger, M. F., Lane, M. C., Loranger, A. W., & Kessler, R. C. (2007). DSM-IV personality disorders in the National Comorbidity Survey Replication. *Biological Psychiatry, 62*(6), 553–564. https://doi.org/10.1016/j.biopsych.2006.09.019

Lilienfeld, S. O., Watts, A. L., & Smith, S. F. (2015). Successful psychopathy: A scientific status report. *Current Directions in Psychological Science, 24*(4), 298–303. https://doi.org/10.1177/0963721415580297

Litten, V., Roberts, L. D., Ladyshewsky, R. K., Castell, E., & Kane, R. (2018). The influence of academic discipline on empathy and psychopathic personality traits in undergraduate students. *Personality and Individual Differences, 123*, 145–150. https://doi.org/10.1016/j.paid.2017.11.025

Litten, V., Roberts, L. D., Ladyshewsky, R. K., Castell, E., & Kane, R. (2020). Empathy and psychopathic traits as predictors of selection into business or psychology disciplines. *Australian Journal of Psychology, 72*(1), 93–105. https://doi.org/10.1111/ajpy.12263

Lochman, J. E., Dishion, T. J., Powell, N. P., Boxmeyer, C. L., Qu, L., & Sallee, M. (2015). Evidence-based preventive intervention for preadolescent aggressive children: One-year outcomes following randomization to group versus individual delivery. *Journal of Consulting and Clinical Psychology, 83*(4), 728–735. https://doi.org/10.1037/ccp0000030

Lonsway, K. A., & Fitzgerald, L. F. (1994). Rape myths: In review. *Psychology of Women Quarterly, 18*(2), 133–164. https://doi.org/10.1111/j.1471-6402.1994.tb00448.x

Lykken, D. T. (1995). *The antisocial personalities*. Lawrence Erlbaum Associates.

Lynam, D. R. (1996). *Early identification of chronic offenders: Who is the fledgling psychopath?* (p. 26).

Lynam, D. R., Charnigo, R., Moffitt, T. E., Raine, A., Loeber, R., & Stouthamer-Loeber, M. (2009). The stability of psychopathy across adolescence. *Development and Psychopathology, 21*(4), 1133. https://doi.org/10.1017/S0954579409990083

McMahon, R. J., Wells, K. C., & Kotler, J. S. (2006). Conduct problems. In E. J. Mash & R. A. Barkley (Eds.), *Treatment of childhood disorders* (pp. 137–268). The Guilford Press.

Mouilso, E. R., & Calhoun, K. S. (2013). The role of rape myth acceptance and psychopathy in sexual assault perpetration. *Journal of Aggression, Maltreatment & Trauma, 22*(2), 159–174. https://doi.org/10.1080/10926771.2013.743937

Mullins-Nelson, J. L., Salekin, R. T., & Leistico, A.-M. R. (2006). Psychopathy, empathy, and perspective -taking ability in a community sample: Implications for the successful psychopathy concept. *International Journal of Forensic Mental Health, 5*(2), 133–149. https://doi.org/1 0.1080/14999013.2006.10471238

O'Connell, D., & Marcus, D. K. (2016). Psychopathic personality traits predict positive attitudes toward sexually predatory behaviors in college men and women. *Personality and Individual Differences, 94*, 372–376. https://doi.org/10.1016/j.paid.2016.02.011

Paulhus, D. L., & Dubois, P. J. (2015). The link between cognitive ability and scholastic cheating: A meta-analysis. *Review of General Psychology, 19*(2), 183–190. https://doi.org/10.1037/ gpr0000040

Payne, D., Lonsway, K., & Fitzgerald, F. (1994). Rape myth acceptance: Exploration of its structure and its measurement using the Illinois rape myth acceptance scale. *Journal of Research in Personality, 33*(1), 27–68. https://doi.org/10.1006/jrpe.1998.2238

Perry, C. (2015). The "dark traits" of sociopathic leaders: Could they be a threat to universities? *The Australian Universities' review, 57*, 17–25.

Pheko, M. M. (2018). Rumors and gossip as tools of social undermining and social dominance in workplace bullying and mobbing practices: A closer look at perceived perpetrator motives. *Journal of Human Behavior in the Social Environment, 28*(4), 449–465. https://doi.org/10.108 0/10911359.2017.1421111

Pisano, S., Muratori, P., Gorga, C., Levantini, V., Iuliano, R., Catone, G., Coppola, G., Milone, A., & Masi, G. (2017). Conduct disorders and psychopathy in children and adolescents: Aetiology, clinical presentation and treatment strategies of callous-unemotional traits. *Italian Journal of Pediatrics, 43*(1), 84. https://doi.org/10.1186/s13052-017-0404-6

Ragatz, L. L., Anderson, R. J., Fremouw, W., & Schwartz, R. (2011). Criminal thinking patterns, aggression styles, and the psychopathic traits of late high school bullies and bully-victims. *Aggressive Behavior, 37*(2), 145–160. https://doi.org/10.1002/ab.20377

Ray, J. V., Poythress, N. G., Weir, J. M., & Rickelm, A. (2009). Relationships between psychopathy and impulsivity in the domain of self-reported personality features. *Personality and Individual Differences, 46*(2), 83–87. https://doi.org/10.1016/j.paid.2008.09.005.

Ribeiro da Silva, D., Rijo, D., & Salekin, R. T. (2020). Psychopathic traits in children and youth: The state-of-the-art after 30 years of research. *Aggression and Violent Behavior, 55*, 101454. https://doi.org/10.1016/j.avb.2020.101454

Sekhar, S., Uppal, N., & Shukla, A. (2020). Dispositional greed and its dark allies: An investigation among prospective managers. *Personality and Individual Differences, 162*, 110005. https://doi. org/10.1016/j.paid.2020.110005.

Salekin, R. T., & Lynam, D. R. (Eds.). (2010). *Handbook of child and adolescent psychopathy*. Guilford Press.

Sellbom, M., & Drislane, L. E. (2020). The classification of psychopathy. *Aggression and Violent Behavior, 101473*. https://doi.org/10.1016/j.avb.2020.101473

Skeem, J. L., Polaschek, D. L. L., Patrick, C. J., & Lilienfeld, S. O. (2011). Psychopathic personality: Bridging the gap between scientific evidence and public policy. *Psychological Science in the Public Interest, 12*(3), 95–162. https://doi.org/10.1177/1529100611426706.

Trull, T. J., Jahng, S., Tomko, R. L., Wood, P. K., & Sher, K. J. (2010). Revised NESARC personality disorder diagnoses: Gender, prevalence, and comorbidity with substance dependence disorders. *Journal of Personality Disorders, 24*(4), 412–426. https://doi.org/10.1521/pedi.2010.24.4.412

Vaughn, M. G., DeLisi, M., Beaver, K. M., Wexler, J., Barth, A., & Fletcher, J. (2010). Juvenile psychopathic personality traits are associated with poor reading achievement. *Psychiatric Quarterly, 82*(3), 177–190. http://dx.doi.org.ezproxylocal.library.nova.edu/10.1007/s11126-010-9162-y

Vedel, A., & Thomsen, D. K. (2017). The dark triad across academic majors. *Personality and Individual Differences, 116*, 86–91. https://doi.org/10.1016/j.paid.2017.04.030

Waller, R., Gardner, F., & Hyde, L. W. (2013). What are the associations between parenting, callous–unemotional traits, and antisocial behavior in youth? A systematic review of evidence. *Clinical Psychology Review, 33*(4), 593–608. https://doi.org/10.1016/j.cpr.2013.03.001

Walsh, J. A., Krienert, J. L., Thresher, G., & Potratz, K. (2018). Examining the link between bullying participation, psychopathy and empathy in a large retrospective sample of university students. *Criminal Justice Studies, 31*(3), 249–266. https://doi.org/10.1080/1478601X.2018.1461625

Watts, A. L., Bowes, S. M., Latzman, R. D., & Lilienfeld, S. O. (2017). Psychopathic traits predict harsh attitudes toward rape victims among undergraduates. *Personality and Individual Differences, 106*, 1–5. https://doi.org/10.1016/j.paid.2016.10.022

Weiler, B. L., & Widom, C. S. (1996). Psychopathy and violent behaviour in abused and neglected young adults. *Criminal Behaviour and Mental Health, 6*(3), 253–271. https://doi.org/10.1002/cbm.99

Widom, C. S. (1977). A methodology for studying noninstitutionalized psychopaths. *Journal of Consulting and Clinical Psychology, 45*(4), 674–683.

Wilkinson, S., Waller, R., & Viding, E. (2016). Practitioner review: Involving young people with callous unemotional traits in treatment – does it work? A systematic review. *Journal of Child Psychology and Psychiatry, 57*(5), 552–565. https://doi.org/10.1111/jcpp.12494

Williams, K. M., Nathanson, C., & Paulhus, D. L. (2010). Identifying and profiling scholastic cheaters: Their personality, cognitive ability, and motivation. *Journal of Experimental Psychology: Applied, 16*(3), 293–307. https://doi.org/10.1037/a0020773

Wilson, M. S., & McCarthy, K. (2011). Greed is good? Student disciplinary choice and self-reported psychopathy. *Personality and Individual Differences, 51*(7), 873–876. https://doi.org/10.1016/j.paid.2011.07.028

Chapter 6
Corporate

6.1 Introduction

First introduced in the book, "Mask of Sanity" by Cleckley (1941), the corporate psychopath—otherwise known as successful, industrial, executive, and organizational psychopath (Boddy, 2014)—has captured the attention of researchers and the general population. Growing interest in this subject has driven researchers to examine the paradox of "successful" psychopathy. In psychopathy literature, "success" does not have a singular connotation, and studies have operationalized "success" as professional achievement, amassing great wealth, celebrity (albeit this fame may be due to some level of notoriety), prosocial behaviors (Skeem et al., 2011), or simply not living in a correctional setting (Lilienfeld et al., 2016). On the other hand, "unsuccessful" psychopaths are commonly seen as individuals who are unable or unwilling to live within societal norms and become involved in criminal behavior that results in incarceration (Benning et al., 2018). Within this dichotomy of "successful" versus "unsuccessful" psychopathy, corporate psychopaths may be a subcategory of the successful type. Popular psychology and works of fiction have fed misconceptions regarding the prevalence and presentations of these individuals (Lilienfeld et al., 2016). This fascination with corporate psychopaths has seemingly fueled listicles and media that purport how a bad boss or rude coworker could be a psychopath in disguise (e.g., *How To Tell If You Work For A Sociopath Or Psychopath* (Kelly, 2019), *20 Signs That Your Boss May Be a Psychopath* (Whitbourne, 2015); *15 Signs Your Boss Is a Psychopath* (Greenwald, 2018); *15 signs your coworker is a psychopath* (Cain, 2017)). While some articles responsibly present disclaimers regarding diagnosis and overgeneralization of psychopathy, boiling workplace psychopathy down to an easily digestible list can be problematic. As these representations are often limiting and do not capture the nature or complexity of psychopathy in the workplace (Landay et al., 2018). In actuality, corporate psychopaths encompass a range of maladaptive behaviors and a constellation of psychopathic traits

T. D. Kennedy et al., *Working with Psychopathy*, SpringerBriefs in Psychology,
https://doi.org/10.1007/978-3-030-84025-9_6

which may or may not completely adhere to the current conceptualization of psychopathy (Sellbom & Drislane, 2020). Which begs the question, who are corporate psychopaths?

The current body of literature primarily focuses on psychopathy within forensic settings (e.g., correctional facilities), but there is less empirical research regarding psychopathy in the corporate world. Therefore, much of the application and scientific understanding regarding psychopaths is based on criminal populations (Benning et al., 2018). From a societal perspective, psychopathy has become synonymous with criminality, in part because "unsuccessful" psychopaths within forensic populations that act in extremes are more likely to gain media attention, specifically when it comes to violence (Edens, 2006). It is important to note that corporate psychopaths may still engage in committing criminal acts (Perri, 2011; Perri, 2013; Boddy et al., 2015). However, even though corporate psychopaths are more likely to commit crime than the general public, their criminal behavior is more closely associated with white-collar crimes, such as fraud (Ragatz et al., 2012), rather than violent offending (Boddy et al., 2015). Psychopathy is considered a risk factor for white-collar crimes, but this link requires further investigation (Perri, 2011). More importantly, this population is not solely defined by their association with criminality. To the contrary, corporate psychopaths are capable of operating within legal boundaries, the impacts of their behaviors are often covert, having a wide range of effects on colleagues, clients, and their business as a whole (Boddy, 2011a).

Much of the research regarding corporate psychopaths centers around leadership (e.g., Boddy, 2011a; Boddy et al., 2015; Boddy, 2017; Landay et al., 2018; Mathieu et al., 2013; Spencer & Byrne, 2016). Some researchers examining the "dark side" of leadership have indicated how problematic leadership styles can negatively impact the workplace (Mathieu et al., 2014). Many of the negative traits associated with "dark leadership" are attributed to individual personality characteristics which ultimately influence employee outcomes (Mathieu et al., 2014), profit margins, and productivity (Boddy, 2014). Because psychopathic traits are variable from one individual to the next (Sellbom & Drislane, 2020), less extreme or covert behaviors may be difficult to detect.

6.2 Prevalence

The prevalence of psychopathy has been estimated at 0.5–1% of the general population; unfortunately, there is no consensus in the literature regarding the presence of these individuals in the workplace. A study by Babiak et al. (2010) identified a higher prevalence of psychopathy within a corporate setting, and their results indicated approximately 4% of high-level managers were psychopaths. In contrast, research by Boddy (2011a) evaluating the correlation between workplace bullying and psychopathic supervisors found that of the 346 white-collar employees in the sample, 5.75% currently had a psychopathic manager, and 32.1% reported having a psychopathic manager at one point in their careers.

6.3 Theoretical Models

While corporate psychopaths share similarities to their "unsuccessful" counterparts, research has indicated several key differences. Three major models regarding successful psychopaths have emerged, each attempting to bridge this gap in scientific knowledge (Lilienfeld et al., 2015).

The moderated-expression model proposes that successful psychopaths are more likely to have protective factors that promote socially adaptive behaviors. Successful psychopaths outperformed unsuccessful psychopaths in autonomic responsivity and executive functioning tasks (Ishikawa et al., 2001; Gao et al., 2011; Widom, 1977). These findings suggest that successful psychopaths may have higher levels of intelligence in comparison to psychopaths deemed as unsuccessful. Intelligence may also contribute to an overall reduction in antisocial behaviors (Wall et al., 2013). Additionally, some research has found that children with psychopathic tendencies such as callous- unemotional traits are more responsive to positive parental styles which incorporate warmth and positive reinforcement (Frick & White, 2008; Waller et al., 2013). These parental factors may lead to positive changes in the development and presentation of psychopathy later in life (Lykken, 1995).

The differential-severity model identifies psychopathy as a singular construct which exists on a continuum of severity. This model theorizes that the primary difference in successful and unsuccessful psychopaths is the level of severity that psychopathic traits are expressed. Research conducted by Ishikawa and colleagues (2001) began by identifying psychopathy using the Psychopathy Checklist-Revised (PCL-R), and the participants were then categorized as either successful or unsuccessful based on criminal conviction histories. Participants predominantly varied on Factor 2 of the PCL-R, indicating that unsuccessful psychopaths are more likely to exhibit antisocial behavior. However, participants did not differ in Factor 1 which is comprised of aspect of personality, such as superficial charm, lack of empathy, etc., that are fundamental to psychopathy (Ishikawa et al., 2001).

The differential-configuration model proposes that successful psychopaths have personality traits that contribute to their success. Differential configuration aligns with the conceptualization that psychopathy is a constellation of characteristics rooted in the three dimensions of the triarchic model, boldness, disinhibition, and meanness (Patrick et al., 2009; see Recognizing a psychopath: Conceptual confusion, 2.4 Triarchic Psychopathy Measure: TriPM). Lilienfeld et al. (2015) suggest "successful" psychopaths likely exhibit the high boldness, low disinhibition, and meanness. Theoretically, boldness may be higher in "successful" in comparison to "unsuccessful" psychopaths (Patrick et al., 2009; Lilienfeld et al., 2016; Persson & Lilienfeld, 2019). Additionally, boldness and low disinhibition have been linked to adaptive functioning (Persson & Lilienfeld, 2019).

6.4   Assessment

The Psychopathy Checklist-Revised (PCL-R) has been widely used in psychopathy evaluation (Mathieu & Babiak, 2016). The PCL-R is an interview-based assessment that was originally created and normed on forensic populations but has demonstrated utility in a variety of clinical settings as well (Hare, 1996; Hare & Neumann, 2008). However, with the recent surge in corporate psychopathy research, there has been a push to create and validate measures specifically designed for use in business settings. Additionally, Mathieu and Babiak (2016) argue that interview-based assessments may be intrusive and typically require specialized training for their administration. While various measures of psychopathy exist, we aim to highlight two promising business-focused measures that provide an opportunity for assessment using multiple reporters.

To address the lack of corporate-specific psychopathy measures, researchers constructed the Business-Scan Self (Mathieu & Babiak, 2016) and the Business-Scan 360 (Mathieu et al., 2013). The two B-Scan iterations primarily differ on the reporter, the 360 version is an employee rating of direct supervisors, and the self-version is based on the self-report of an individual. Both of the B-Scan assessments are based on the PCL-R four-factor structural model (Mathieu et al., 2013; Mathieu & Babiak, 2016). The B-Scan 360 is a 20-item, Likert scale questionnaire assessing employees' perceptions of personality (i.e., psychopathy) in their direct supervisors. Similarly, the B-Scan Self is currently a 60-item self-report, Likert scale questionnaire, created to assess psychopathic traits of an individual (Mathieu & Babiak, 2016).

To identify the factor structure of the B-Scan 360, Mathieu et al. (2013) implemented a two-part study. The first study used an exploratory analysis of 340 adult employees, to discern the factor structure to be used based on the original 113 items. The results of this analysis identified 20 equally distributed items that loaded onto the following four factors: Manipulative/Unethical, Callous/Insensitive, Unreliable/Unfocused, and Intimidating/Aggressive. Next using confirmatory factor analysis (CFA), the authors utilized a new sample of 806 adult employees to test the model. The results of the CFA found acceptable fit for the model, with similar levels of reliability when compared to the exploratory analysis (Mathieu et al., 2013).

Mathieu and Babiak (2016) later developed the B-Scan Self as a means of assessing self-reported psychopathic traits of individuals in business settings. Items for the B-Scan Self were adapted from the B-Scan 360, to reflect a self-report style questionnaire. The initial part of the study was conducted with 514 adults, using confirmatory factor analysis (CFA) to validate the four-factor structure and 15 facets of the B-Scan Self model. The results indicated the 15 facets acceptably load onto the four-factor structure (i.e., Interpersonal, Affective, Lifestyle, and Antisocial). The Interpersonal factor contains four facets: insincere, arrogant, untrustworthy, and manipulative/unethical. In the Affective factor, four facets are present: remorseless, shallow, insensitive, and blaming. There are five facets that comprise the Lifestyle factor: impatient, selfish, unfocused, erratic, and unreliable. Finally, only two facets are found under the Antisocial factor: bullying and dramatic. A second-order CFA was conducted utilizing a second sample of 397 adults, to assess the final factor structure. Based on the results of both CFAs, authors found an acceptable fit for the four-factor model and 15 facets of the B-Scan Self (Mathieu & Babiak, 2016).

6.5 Presentation

Attempting to define the presentation of psychopathy is not without its caveats, as previously mentioned psychopathy can be conceptualized as a spectrum including a variety of associated traits. An individual may present differently depending on where they fall on that continuum. The differential expression of psychopathy may vary based on additional factors such as gender and early childhood development (Lykken, 1995; Hicks & Drislane, 2018). Most research regarding corporate psychopaths focuses on business leaders who are high in psychopathic traits (e.g., Boddy, 2011a; Mathieu et al., 2014; Boddy, 2015a, 2015b). Significantly less research has investigated the presence or effects of psychopathic subordinates in the workplace (e.g., Hurst et al., 2019).

The literature has identified several commonalities and trends employed by these individuals in the business realm. A qualitative study conducted by Boddy et al. (2015) revealed psychopathic management styles tend to exhibit striking similarities. For instance, corporate psychopaths overwhelmingly utilized intimidation, coercion, and threats which foster extreme work environments. These overt behaviors are also utilized to cause conflict and confusion and promote fear within these environments (Clarke, 2005; Hare, 1999). Those with psychopathic traits often employ a toolbox for managing their environments complete with both overt and covert implements (Babiak & Hare, 2006). In practice, the identification of individuals with psychopathic traits in the workplace is challenging, as many corporate psychopaths tend to obfuscate their personal behavior and goals through covert manipulative tactics (Babiak & Hare, 2006; Babiak, 2000). In the long term, these manipulative tactics often come to light, and the psychopath is exposed (Babiak & Hare, 2006). However, in extreme environments where poor communication and distrust are rampant, exposure does not always result in the removal of the psychopath (Boddy et al., 2015). Skilled psychopathic manipulators can utilize prudent planning and strategic positioning to gain access to higher level positions regardless of negative appraisals by others (Babiak, 2000). These extreme environments may be identified by high turnover rates, low employee satisfaction, and a lack of communication within and between departments (Boddy et al., 2015).

6.5.1 Dysfunctional Versus Psychopathic

Other issues arise when attempting to disentangle the behavior of dysfunctional versus psychopathic leaders. Dysfunctional leaders are described in the literature as individuals in managerial positions who have psychopathic traits but who do not fully meet criteria for psychopathy (Boddy, 2011a) and individuals in positions of power whose behavior causes impediments to the "operational function" at any level of the corporate hierarchy (Rose et al., 2015). Dysfunctional leaders tend to exhibit similar maladaptive management styles when compared to psychopathic leaders including bullying, intimidation, lying, and overt displays of aggression (e.g., yelling; Boddy, 2011a; Boddy et al., 2015; Rose et al., 2015). What sets corporate psychopaths apart is the frequency and intensity of these maladaptive behaviors (Boddy, 2011a) combined with their mask of superficial charms (Hare, 1999). Notably, charm alone is not inherently a dishonest display to socially manipulate others to form a positive impression. In the context of psychopathy, charm should be evaluated based on intention. Psychopathic charm is a self-serving means to an end. Furthermore, its implementation comes with a level of callousness and intentional disregard for others (Babiak & Hare, 2006).

6.5.2   Manipulation

Manipulation encompasses a range of tactics employed by psychopaths to control others (Babiak & Hare, 2006; Babiak, 2000). For example, impression management is a form of manipulation that is used by psychopaths to intentionally misrepresent themselves or situations to for their own benefit. Impression management is commonly utilized as a method of reformulating the narrative surrounding negative behavior and personal failings, thus controlling perceptions of higher-ups. As described in *Snakes in Suits: When Psychopaths go to Work* by Babiak and Hare (2006), in predatory manipulation, a large segment of psychopaths make use of the "three-phase process" comprised of assessment, manipulation, and abandonment. In the assessment phase, psychopaths will gauge an individual's worth in relation to themselves, essentially determining how useful the target might be. From a corporate standpoint, those with influence and power are particularly enticing targets (e.g., high-level executives). It is important to note that targets are not limited to higher-ups, and indirect or "informal power" might include low-level employees who carry special influence in the workplace. Throughout this phase, the psychopath will evaluate emotional vulnerabilities, looking for weaknesses to exploit. During the manipulation phase, psychopaths will use what they have learned during their assessment to customize their manipulations. Psychopaths will tailor their presentation, procuring an effective façade to garner trust. Lying is engrained in their interactions and is often calculated and instrumental to their manipulation. When caught in a lie, psychopaths may alter their deceptions to be more believable or resort to gaslighting (i.e., psychological abuse in the form of challenging a person's memory or perception of reality) their victims. The ultimate goal is to gain something from their target. Finally, abandonment occurs once the psychopath has exhausted their victim's usefulness, and they will move on (Babiak & Hare, 2006).

The psychopathic process model provides a similar explanation for psychopathic manipulation but at a corporate level. This 5-phase model focuses on career stages commonly seen in workplace psychopathy, including organizational entry, assessment, manipulation, confrontation, and ascension (Babiak, 2000). The organizational entry phase covers the hiring process, where psychopaths utilize their superficial charms to game the system. Frequently, psychopaths tend to exaggerate or fabricate their qualifications. As psychopaths are often adept at persuading others of their knowledge and abilities, unsuspecting interviewers may have difficulties ascertaining the true quality of potential job candidates. After a psychopath has been hired, they will enter the assessment phase, identifying important people and how to use them, evaluating interpersonal relations between coworkers as well as the company ethos. The manipulation phase resembles a metaphorical hostile takeover of workplace communications, where the psychopath turns the workplace into their own personal data mine, simultaneously spreading lies to benefit themselves as much as possible. The purpose of these curated communications is to bolster the psychopath's reputation and sow discord among their colleagues. The confrontation phase occurs when the psychopath's victims start to recognize they have been taken advantage of. Although the maladaptive behaviors and abuses they have endured have become apparent, victims may have no place to turn because the psychopath has effectively defused these prospective malcontents through the spread of disinformation. Additionally, confrontation may also come about indirectly, resulting from people they have used and abandoned seeking the comfort of others and sharing their experiences. The final stage of this process is the ascension phase, whereby the psychopath utilizes the groundwork laid out during the four previous phases to move up within the company. This can be accomplished by scapegoating the "patrons" who have been shielding the psychopath from negative repercussions until this point (Babiak, 2000).

6.5.3   Bullying

One of the most common forms of overt behaviors is workplace bullying. Boddy (2011a) describes bullying as "the repeated unethical and unfavorable treatment of one person by another in the workplace" (p. 367). Bullying is more frequent in high demand jobs where power differentials are at play. Research has found the majority of bullying is associated with a minority of leaders (Boddy, 2011a; Boddy, 2014). For instance, corporate psychopaths made up approximately 1% of the workforce but were found to be disproportionately responsible for 26% of bullying (Boddy, 2011a). Another study found psychopaths are accountable for approximately 35% of workplace bullying (Boddy, 2014). Notably, Boddy and Taplin (2017) suggest that previous studies may have underestimated the prevalence of workplace bullying perpetrated by corporate psychopaths. Previously used bullying measures potentially lacked adequate sensitivity to accurately assess the frequency or severity of these behaviors (Boddy & Taplin, 2017).

Bullying can manifest in a variety of ways, such as intentional humiliation, insinuations of job insecurity, outright threats to job safety, intimidation, abusive language, yelling and beratement (Harvey et al., 2007; Boddy, 2011a; Pheko, 2018).

Garnering some level of acceptance for this type of behavior can be accomplished by manipulation (e.g., turning others against their targets, lying, spreading gossip) and the creation of toxic work environments (Babiak, 2000; Pheko, 2018).

6.5.4   Violence

Criminality for corporate psychopaths frequently takes the form white-collar crime. However, psychopathic behavior may escalate to include violent threats (Boddy et al., 2015) and physical violence (Perri & Lichtenwald, 2010; Perri, 2011). Threats of violence have been reported as a method of control used by psychopathic bosses during employee interviews (Boddy et al., 2015). Physical violence is more of a rarity for corporate psychopaths and may be used as a last resort when other forms of control fail (Perri & Lichtenwald, 2010). Violence in this case is often instrumental, as many of the homicides committed by white-collar criminals were implemented to avoid fraud detection (Perri, 2011).

6.6   Myths and Common Misconceptions

6.6.1   Fictional Representations of Psychopathy

While successful psychopaths are broadly defined in the scientific literature, societal perceptions of psychopaths in the workplace are regularly skewed by sensationalistic and often conflictual information regarding their prevalence and characteristics (Smith & Lilienfeld, 2013; Lilienfeld et al., 2016). To unravel why perceptions of psychopathy are often misguided, it is important to look at representation and exposure. Media popularizations of the psychopathic serial killer have driven public attention to extreme portrayals of psychopathy. Typically, people are more likely to be exposed to versions of psychopathic individuals who have been packaged as devious delinquents and monstrous murderers in fiction or news media, rather than peer-reviewed scientific articles (Skeem et al., 2011). The onus for factual representations of psychopathy does not fall on authors of fiction. However, the mythology surrounding psychopathy is widely derived from combinations of fiction, documentaries, news articles, and scientific half-truths propagated in pop psychology (Skeem et al., 2011). A study by Davis and colleagues (2020) evaluated 24 characters using the two-factor PCL-R model. The authors found only 21% of the psychopathic representations in film met criteria for psychopathy (Davis et al., 2020). For example, one of the most well-known fictional characterizations of corporate psychopathy is Patrick Bateman from the 2000 film, *American Psycho*. As with many representations of psychopathy in modern media, Bateman's depiction is more so an amalgam of mental illnesses rather than a true portrayal of psychopathy. When Bateman is initially introduced, he appears to have all the superficial charm and glibness of a psychopath accompanied by a lack of empathy and methodical application of control. However, as the film reaches its second act, the audience bears witness to Bateman's descent into madness, portrayed as psychosis, namely, hallucinations, delusions, and an insatiable blood lust (Harron, 2000). While fictional film characterizations are one facet of popular media, these depictions give important insights into the proliferation of misinformation consumed by the general public.

6.6.2 Myth of Financial Prowess

Popular representations of psychopath coupled with a lack of conceptual consensus have led to several myths and misconceptions surrounding corporate psychopaths. One of the broader beliefs is that psychopathic individuals can be financially beneficial to companies, especially those that involve high-risk, high- demand work environments (e.g., Wall Street). An article by ten Brinke et al. (2018) investigated the long-term returns of 101 hedge fund managers from 2005 to 2015. Their research indicated that leaders high in psychopathic tendencies demonstrated a slight but significant reduction in annual returns, approximately 1%. Although the percentage may appear low, over a ten-year time frame large investments stand to lose thousands of dollars (ten Brink et al., 2018). Similar results were found by Omar et al. (2019), and psychopathic tendencies were correlated with reduced annual returns. Importantly, the study did not use a formal psychopathy measure; instead a linguistic analysis of annual reports was utilized as a proxy for psychopathic tendencies among management teams and senior leaders (Omar et al., 2019). These differences in returns may be attributable to increased risk-taking (ten Brinke et al., 2018; Omar et al., 2019). Returns on investments are commonly seen as unpredictable; therefore, losses due to excessively risky behavior may be less apparent to investors (Omar et al., 2019). Generally, risk-taking is a type of impulsive behavior that is considered a key component of psychopathy (Hare, 1999).

6.6.3 Impulsivity and Self-Control

Contrary to traditional models of psychopathy which emphasize high levels of impulsivity as a key component in overt displays of maladaptive psychopathic behavior, such as criminality (Hare, 1999), impulsivity may manifest differently in successful psychopaths (Palmen et al., 2020). When investigating impulsivity as it applies to the five-factor model of personality, Whiteside and Lynam (2001) identified four domains related to impulsive behavior: urgency, a lack of premeditation, a lack of perseverance, and sensation-seeking. Risk-taking is associated with a form of impulsivity that falls into the sensation- seeking domain (Whiteside & Lynam, 2001). The sensation-seeking domain of impulsivity is not inherently maladaptive, and high scorers are characterized as individuals who look to engage in thrilling and novel experiences (which can include dangerous activities; Whiteside & Lynam, 2001). This differentiation of impulsivity is important for corporate psychopathy, because engaging in sensation-seeking is associated with increased functionality in comparison to other forms of impulsivity (Whiteside & Lynam, 2001; Poythress & Hall, 2011). According to a model proposed by Palmen et al. (2020), the defining characteristic between "successful" and "unsuccessful" psychopaths may be self-control. On the surface, high self-control and impulsivity are at theoretical odds with one another, but self-control may moderate impulsivity (Palmen et al., 2020; Lasko & Chester, 2020).

Self-control may take the form of increased levels of conscientiousness. Using the five-factor model of personality, Mullins-Sweatt et al. (2010) evaluated 120 "successful" individuals with psychopathic traits, and their findings suggest high levels of contentiousness within this population. In a longitudinal study utilizing reduced recidivism as a marker of comparative success in 1354 adolescent offenders, Lasko and Chester (2020) investigated the relationship between psychopathic grandiose-manipulative traits on the development of increased conscientiousness and impulse control. The results demonstrated that individuals with grandiose-manipulative traits at the onset of the study correlated with success (i.e., reduced recidivism) as well as increased impulse control and conscientiousness. This implies that the regulation of impulsivity could be acquired over time dependent on the differential expression of psychopathic traits (Lasko & Chester, 2020). Honing manipulative skills may subvert the inclination for overt behaviors such as instrumental aggression. Although, conscientiousness does not necessarily insulate individuals from criminal conviction. A study of currently incarcerated business managers found high levels of conscientiousness as a predictor of white-collar crime (Blickle et al., 2006).

6.6.4   Leadership

The notion that those with psychopathic traits are effective managers is another pervasive myth. Psychopathic supervisors contribute to the degradation of employee job satisfaction and emotional well-being, leading to high turnover rates (Boddy, 2014; Boddy et al., 2015; Boddy & Croft, 2016; Boddy, 2017; Omar et al., 2019). A lack of effective management can significantly reduce client satisfaction and damage a company's reputation (Boddy, 2012; Boddy & Croft, 2016). The results of a study conducted by Boddy (2014) suggest that employees working under psychopathic managers are more prone to engage in counterproductive work behavior (i.e., intentionally acting in a manner that will likely result in negative outcomes for the company) as a method of retribution for unfair and malicious treatment. This indirect form of aggression has a negative effect on both *efficiency and productivity*. The presence of psychopathy in the workplace often leads to declining emotional well-being in others. For instance, employees with psychopathic managers are more likely to report negative feelings (e.g., anger, boredom) and less likely to endorse positive feelings (e.g., contentment; Boddy, 2014). Job satisfaction is negatively impacted by psychopathic management, and employees may lose a clear sense of purpose and enthusiasm in these workplace environments (Boddy, 2017). A qualitative case study conducted by Boddy and Croft (2016) followed the effects of marketing function in two companies, each lead by an ineffectual psychopathic CEO or director. Both organizations reported sharp decreases in employee and customer satisfaction, as well as significant employee loss. One manager noted a 100% turnover rate within a two-year period due to problematic leadership (Boddy & Croft, 2016). On the other hand, research by Spencer and Byrne (2016) indicated employees did not differ on job satisfaction based on the presence of psychopathic supervisors. However, as discussed in the limitations, only 54.9% of employees were willing to participate which may relate to the presence of bias in the sample (Spencer & Byrne, 2016).

6.7 Adaptive Benefits

6.7.1 Psychopathic Subordinates

Considering psychopathy as adaptive is not without its merits. In a study from Hurst, Simon, Jung, and Pirouz (2019), employees with higher levels of primary psychopathy were more likely to thrive in abusive environments when compared to coworkers. Not only were employees with high scores on primary psychopathy less angry under abusive supervision than their non-psychopathic peers, but they also demonstrated increased engagement and positive affect (Hurst et al., 2019). These findings may parallel studies indicating psychopaths are typically less reactive both physiologically (Benning et al., 2005; Blair et al., 2002; Hare et al., 1978) and emotionally (Pletti et al., 2017). Notably, the apparent workplace gains associated with high primary psychopathy dissipate in the presence of non-abusive supervisors (Hurst et al., 2019).

6.7.2 Financial and Entrepreneurial Success

Research conducted by Persson and Lilienfeld (2019) attempted to identify how the three factors of triarchic model (i.e., boldness, meanness, and disinhibition; Patrick et al., 2009) are conceptually linked to successful psychopathy. The authors propose that "high social status" and "a lack of serious antisocial behavior" are both important dimensions of "success" in psychopathy. Notably, this study utilized socioeconomic status (SES) to indicate "high social status." The findings demonstrated boldness was associated with higher SES and less antisocial behaviors. Whereas disinhibition and meanness both corresponded with more antisocial behavior. Disinhibition was also found to correlate negatively with SES (Persson & Lilienfeld, 2019).

An article by Akhtar et al. (2013) found primary psychopathy positively pre-dicted entrepreneurial tendencies and abilities. This result may be due in part to the self-report nature of the assessments, as abilities, tendencies, and success were sus-ceptible to an individual's perceived attributes versus actual competence. As pri-mary psychopathy was only observed to be a modest predictor of entrepreneurial success (Akhtar et al., 2013), this outcome may relate to psychopathic grandiosity. Individuals high in primary psychopathy may perceive themselves as more capable and desirable in a job setting due to grandiosity.

6.7.3   Corporate Entry and Ascension

Psychopathic traits such as superficial charm, grandiosity, and glibness may be ben-eficial during interviews and promotions (Babiak, 2000). Within a corporate struc-ture those high in psychopathic tendencies appear to be more prevalent within the upper levels of management (Spencer & Byrne, 2016). Babiak et al. (2010) report a trend during the hiring stage where high-level managers rely on first impressions and "gut feelings" about job candidates. These initial impressions permeate future perceptions of employee behavior (Pech & Slade, 2007). Therefore, despite com-plaints or poor performance evaluations, higher-ups seemingly engage in a type of confirmation bias that leans heavily on their interpretations (Babiak et al., 2010). As individuals with psychopathic traits often have a flare for manipulation, they are likely to sway the narrative surrounding these events in their favor (Babiak & Hare, 2006; Babiak, 2000). If viewing traditionally psychopathic traits through the dis-torted lens of positive attributions, many of these behaviors could be ascribed to optimum leadership traits (Babiak et al., 2010; Boddy et al., 2015). Despite the exertion of abusive supervision, psychopathic leaders were given high levels of sup-port by their superiors (Boddy et al., 2015).

Importantly, this perceived potential can propel an individual with subpar work performance and dismal interpersonal skills to the upper echelons of corporate enti-ties (Pech & Slade, 2007). However, this outcome is somewhat conditional in nature. Firstly, corporate psychopaths thrive in certain environments where confu-sion, competition, and fear are prevalent (Babiak, 2000; Boddy, 2011b; Boddy et al., 2015). Unstable organizations with high turnover rates (Boddy, 2011b; Boddy, 2014) and low oversite are rife with confusion, creating an optimum environment for psychopathic management (Babiak, 2000). From a capitalistic standpoint, where profit margins are valued over interpersonal skills, an individual's potential for increasing financial gain is regarded as both a rare and essential quality (Boddy, 2011b; Boddy et al., 2015). According to Boddy's Corporate Psychopaths Theory of the Global Financial Crisis, shifts in employment practices have significantly contributed to the increase of corporate psychopaths occupying high-level roles. Therefore, the crisis may have been driven by the unchecked avarice of corporate psychopaths due to their capacity to wield influence (Boddy, 2011b).

6.8 Gender Differences

6.8.1 Differential Expression

In many of the studies that report demographic distributions across samples, corporate leaders are overwhelmingly male (e.g., Babiak et al., 2010; Spencer & Byrne, 2016; ten Brink et al., 2018). Generally, men are overrepresented in psychopathy research (Skeem et al., 2011), in part due to the reliance on forensic samples which are disproportionately male. It is a myth that psychopathy is exclusively male (Berg et al., 2013). Women can also possess psychopathic traits, and some research has suggested a differential in psychopathic behavioral expression between men and women (Verona & Vitale, 2018). One research study indicated that women were more likely to engage in cooperative tasks than men regardless of psychopathic tendencies (Rilling et al., 2007). Additionally, successful female psychopaths are less likely to engage in antisocial behaviors (e.g., criminal behavior) but are more likely to utilize manipulation (Eisenbarth, 2014).

6.8.2 Differential Advantages for Men and Women

Psychopathic traits may not be equally beneficial for women, indicating a potentially gender-based dynamic at play. A metanalysis of 92 studies found male psychopaths in the workplace were more likely to be promoted to leadership roles as well as be seen as effective. On the other hand, the same article identified a negative relationship between female psychopathy and being viewed as an effective leader. Additionally, when compared to men with the same traits, psychopathic females were less likely to be promoted to leadership roles (Landay et al., 2018). An investigation of gender differences in other Dark Triad traits, such as narcissism, has demonstrated similar findings. Narcissistic leaders when evaluated by male subordinates rated women as less effective in comparison to men (De Hoogh et al., 2015). These results may be attributed to perceptions of gender roles perpetuating gender biases in the workplace (Heilman, 2001).

Generally speaking, researchers have found significant gender biases within corporate structures. Hurst and colleagues (2019) theorize that men and women in leadership likely have similar traits; however, women with psychopathic traits are not promoted at similar rates when compared to their male counterparts. In an analysis of promotional considerations for men and women, men are significantly more likely to be promoted based on their potential, where women are typically promoted based on merit (Player et al., 2019). The same holds true for hiring practices. This differential in rewards goes beyond potential versus merit and may even translate into traditional gender roles (Phelan et al., 2008). The rationale may lie in the expectations of male and female behavior and the prevalence of toxic masculinity in male-dominated professions. Toxic masculinity as described by Kupers (2005) "involves the need to aggressively compete and dominate others and encompasses the most problematic proclivities in men" (p. 713). On the surface, toxic masculinity mirrors psychopathic traits. In the workplace, this translates to ideas that men are expected to suppress emotionality, engage in competition, display dominance, and be ambitious. These seemingly traditional male virtues can also negatively impact men who subvert gender roles. In one study, comparing traits of men and women applying for leadership roles (where practical and social aptitude were key components of the position) men were assessed more negatively compared to women, when they presented themselves in a manner that did not conform to traditional gender stereotypes (e.g., having an exceedingly modest disposition; Moss-Racusin et al., 2010). Conversely, women who demonstrated conventionally valued leadership traits among men, such as self-confidence, ambition, and competitive dispositions, were evaluated as less desirable job candidates (Phelan et al. 2008).

6.8.3 Case Study: Elizabeth Holmes

Elizabeth Holmes founder and former CEO of Theranos, a private healthcare and life sciences company, claimed to revolutionize medicine with cutting edge technologies that would forever change the way in which blood tests were collected, processed, and analyzed. According to the inditement (U.S. v. Holmes and Balwani), Elizabeth Holmes and Ramesh Balwani were involved in a multimillion-dollar scheme to defraud investors. They have been charged with nine counts of wire fraud and two counts of conspiracy to commit fraud. Although the upcoming trial and circumstances surrounding the case have been widely publicized, it is important to note these allegations have yet to result in any convictions. She has been accused of making falsified claims surrounding new "cheap and effective" blood testing technology and concealing and manipulating test results to investors during research and development (U.S. v. Holmes and Balwani).

In the book, Bad Blood: Secrets and Lies in a Silicon Valley Startup, Carreyrou (2018) details several cues that Holmes may have psychopathic traits. Holmes reportedly created a false persona, changing her voice and presentation to influence the perception of others. She allegedly misrepresented her knowledge and abilities to gain trust from employees and investors. These behaviors were notably accompanied by grandiose claims that her proposed technologies could "change mankind." Reportedly, she also engaged in blackmail and legal action against former employees of Theranos. Most importantly, Carreyrou claims that Holmes carried out these manipulations and lies without expressing remorse or empathy. While individuals who commit white-collar crime are more likely to display psychopathy and narcissism (Perri, 2011), it is necessary to emphasize, to our knowledge, Holmes has not been formally assessed for psychopathy (Carreyrou, 2018).

6.9 Summary

Corporate psychopaths present an opportunity to better understand psychopathy outside of forensic settings. Based on the research findings, individuals with psychopathic traits in the corporate realm are more likely to be high in primary psychopathy (e.g., superficial charm, shallow affect, grandiosity). In comparison to the secondary psychopathy that is often seen in criminal populations, primary psychopaths are more likely to have adaptive traits that enable them to be more successful (Mullins-Sweatt et al., 2010; Akhtar et al., 2013; Palmen et al., 2020). While success has a relatively broad connotation, in corporate psychopathy research, success is often characterized by career attainment and achievements. Primary psychopathy traits, such as superficial charm, may benefit psychopaths attempting to make a good first impression on hiring managers (Babiak et al., 2010). These initial impressions accompanied by future manipulations likely drive promotional considerations as well (Pech & Slade, 2007).

Manipulation is often a key facet of covert control asserted by psychopaths in corporate entities (Babiak, 2000; Babiak & Hare, 2006; Babiak et al., 2010). Individuals with psychopathic traits are more likely to align themselves with people in power and use manipulation to garner favor (Babiak, 2000). By controlling the perceptions of others, psychopaths can navigate potential backlash from negative feedback and poor performance. When psychopathic manipulation is eventually found out, it often results in the psychopath moving up (Babiak, 2000) or moving on (Babiak & Hare, 2006). The outcome is often dependent on effective groundwork and whether a person or place has expended their perceived usefulness. However, corporate structures that are permissive of abuse, have poor communication, lack oversight and are unstable, may be more vulnerable to the effects of psychopaths in the workplace (Babiak, 2000).

Employing leaders with psychopathic traits often leads to negative outcomes for clients, employees, and corporate entities. As a whole, leaders high in psychopathic traits are more likely to be abusive to their subordinates (Boddy, 2014; Boddy & Croft, 2016). When these leaders are present, there are more reports by employees of bullying, intimidation, and coercion (Harvey et al., 2007; Boddy, 2011a, 2011b; Pheko, 2018). This can lead to high turnover rates, degrading employee satisfaction (Boddy, 2014; Boddy et al., 2015; Boddy & Croft, 2016; Boddy, 2017; Omar et al., 2019), and counterproductive work behaviors by dispirited employees (Boddy, 2014). When psychopathic leaders are unable to control their colleagues, they may resort to vicious threats or violence (Boddy et al., 2015). Furthermore, psychopaths are more inclined to cause a decline in client satisfaction (Boddy & Croft, 2016), namely, through mismanagement or shear incompetence (Boddy et al., 2015). As psychopaths commonly misrepresent their skills and abilities, it is possible for them to be promoted to a position they are not qualified for (Pech & Slade, 2007). Potentially poor leadership skill sets coupled with maladaptive workplace behavior likely contribute to declines in productivity and corporate profit margins (Boddy, 2014).

Despite clear interpersonal deficits, psychopathic traits are associated with some advantages. Importantly, these advantageous may be limited to male psychopaths, as women who demonstrate these qualities do not seem to benefit equally. In comparison to men, women displaying psychopathic traits are less likely to be promoted or seen as effective leaders (Landay et al., 2018). Knowledge surrounding psychopathic traits in women within the workplace is limited (Hurst et al., 2019). Future research should focus on differential presentations and advantage of gender in corporate psychopathy.

This chapter provides a brief insight into the current body of knowledge regarding corporate psychopathy. Unfortunately, the literature lacks consensus over the conceptualization and manifestations of psychopathy in the workplace (Lilienfeld et al., 2015). However, the present academic findings may provide useful insights for individuals who may encounter corporate psychopaths within the business realm. It is imperative that researchers continue to pursue understanding of psychopathic traits as they relate to the corporate world.

References

Akhtar, R., Ahmetoglu, G., & Chamorro-Premuzic, T. (2013). Greed is good? Assessing the relationship between entrepreneurship and subclinical psychopathy. *Personality and Individual Differences, 54*(3), 420–425. https://doi.org/10.1016/j.paid.2012.10.013

Babiak, P. (2000). Psychopathic manipulation at work. In C. B. Gacono (Ed.), *Personality and clinical psychology series. The clinical and forensic assessment of psychopathy: A practitioner's guide* (pp. 353–373). Routledge/Taylor & Francis Group.

Babiak, P., & Hare, R. D. (2006). *Snakes in suits: When psychopaths go to work*. Regan Books.

Babiak, P., Neumann, C. S., & Hare, R. D. (2010). Corporate psychopathy: Talking the walk. *Behavioral Sciences & the Law.* https://doi.org/10.1002/bsl.925

Benning, S. D., Patrick, C. J., Blonigen, D. M., Hicks, B. M., & Iacono, W. G. (2005). Estimating facets of psychopathy from normal personality traits: A step toward community epidemiological investigations. *Assessment, 12*(1), 3–18. https://doi.org/10.1177/1073191104271223

Benning, S. D., Venables, N. C., & Hall, J. R. (2018). Successful psychopathy. In C. J. Patrick (Ed.), *Handbook of psychopathy* (pp. 585–608). The Guilford Press.

Berg, J. M., Smith, S. F., Watts, A. L., Ammirati, R., Green, S. E., & Lilienfeld, S. O. (2013). Misconceptions regarding psychopathic personality: Implications for clinical practice and research. *Neuropsychiatry, 3*(1), 63–74. https://doi.org/10.2217/npy.12.69

Blair, R. J., Mitchell, D. G., Richell, R. A., Kelly, S., Leonard, A., Newman, C., & Scott, S. K. (2002). Turning a deaf ear to fear: Impaired recognition of vocal affect in psychopathic individuals. *Journal of Abnormal Psychology, 111*(4), 682–686. https://doi.org/10.1037//0021-843x.111.4.682

Blickle, G., Schlegel, A., Fassbender, P., & Klein, U. (2006). Some personality correlates of business white-collar crime. *Applied Psychology, 55*(2), 220–233. https://doi.org/10.1111/j.1464-0597.2006.00226.x

Boddy, C. R. (2011a). Corporate psychopaths, bullying and unfair supervision in the workplace. *Journal of Business Ethics, 100*(3), 367–379. https://doi.org/10.1007/s10551-010-0689-5

Boddy, C. R. (2011b). The corporate psychopaths theory of the global financial crisis. *Journal of Business Ethics, 102*(2), 255–259. https://doi.org/10.1007/s10551-011-0810-4

Boddy, C. (2012). The impact of corporate psychopaths on corporate reputation and marketing. *The Marketing Review, 12*(1). https://doi.org/10.1362/146934712X13286274424343

Boddy, C. R. (2014). Corporate psychopaths, conflict, employee affective well-being and counterproductive work behaviour. *Journal of Business Ethics, 121*(1), 107–121. https://doi.org/10.1007/s10551-013-1688-0

Boddy, C. R. (2015a). Corporate psychopaths: Uncaring citizens, irresponsible leaders. In *Globalization and corporate citizenship: The alternative gaze a collection of seminal essays* (1st ed., pp. 166–177). Greenleaf Publishing Limited. https://doi.org/10.9774/GLEAF.9781783535026_14

Boddy, C. R. (2015b). Organisational psychopaths: A ten year update. *Management Decision, 53*(10), 2407–2432. https://doi.org/10.1108/MD-04-2015-0114

Boddy, C. R. (2017). Psychopathic leadership a case study of a corporate psychopath CEO. *Journal of Business Ethics, 145*(1), 141–156. https://doi.org/10.1007/s10551-015-2908-6

Boddy, C. R., & Croft, R. (2016). Marketing in a time of toxic leadership. *Qualitative Market Research: An International Journal, 19*(1), 44–64. https://doi.org/10.1108/QMR-04-2015-0030

Boddy, C., & Taplin, R. (2017). A note on workplace psychopathic bullying – Measuring its frequency and severity. *Aggression and Violent Behavior, 34*, 117–119. https://doi.org/10.1016/j.avb.2017.02.001

Boddy, C., Miles, D., Sanyal, C., & Hartog, M. (2015). Extreme managers, extreme workplaces: Capitalism, organizations and corporate psychopaths. *Organization, 22*(4), 530–551. https://doi.org/10.1177/1350508415572508

Cain, A. (2017, November 28). *15 signs your coworker is a psychopath.* Business Insider. https://www.businessinsider.com/signs-you-are-working-with-a-psychopath-2017-6

Carreyrou, J. (2018). *Bad Blood: Secrets and Lies in a Silicone Valley Startup.* Vintage Books.

Clarke, J. (2005). *Working with monsters. How to identify and protect yourself from the workplace psychopath.* Random House.

Cleckley, H. (1941). *The mask of sanity: An attempt to reinterpret the so-called psychopathic personality.* Mosby.

Davis, K. M., Frederick, A., & Corcoran, A. (2020). Using the Psychopathy Checklist to examine cinematic portrayals of psychopaths. *Aggression and violent behavior, 52*, 101424. https://doi.org/10.1016/j.avb.2020.101424.

De Hoogh, A. H., Den Hartog, D. N., & Nevicka, B. (2015). Gender differences in the perceived effectiveness of narcissistic leaders. *Applied Psychology, 64*(3), 473–498. https://doi.org/10.1111/apps.12015

Edens, J. F. (2006). Unresolved controversies concerning psychopathy: Implications for clinical and forensic decision making. *Professional Psychology: Research and Practice, 37*(1), 59–65. https://doi.org/10.1037/0735-7028.37.1.59

Eisenbarth, H. (2014). Psychopathic personality in women. Diagnostics and experimental findings in the forensic setting and the business world. *Der Nervenarzt, 85*(3), 290, 292–294, 296–297. http://dx.doi.org.ezproxylocal.library.nova.edu/10.1007/s00115-013-3902-9

Frick, P. J., & White, S. F. (2008). Research review: The importance of callous-unemotional traits for developmental models of aggressive and antisocial behavior. *Journal of Child Psychology and Psychiatry, and Allied Disciplines, 49*(4), 359–375. https://doi.org/10.1111/j.1469-7610.2007.01862.x

Gao, Y., Raine, A., & Schug, R. A. (2011). P3 event-related potentials and childhood maltreatment in successful and unsuccessful psychopaths. *Brain and Cognition, 77*(2), 176–182. https://doi.org/10.1016/j.bandc.2011.06.010

Greenwald, M. (2018, July 12). *15 signs your boss is a psychopath.* Best Life. https://bestlifeonline.com/horrible-bosses/

Hare, R. D. (1996). Psychopathy: A clinical construct whose time has come. *Criminal Justice and Behavior, 23*(1), 25–54. https://doi.org/10.1177/0093854896023001004

Hare, R. (1999). *Without conscience: The disturbing word of the psychopaths among us.* Guildford Press.

Hare, R. D., & Neumann, C. S. (2008). Psychopathy as a clinical and empirical construct. *Annual Review of Clinical Psychology, 4*, 217–246. https://doi.org/10.1146/annurev.clinpsy.3.022806.091452

Hare, R. D., Frazelle, J., & Cox, D. N. (1978). Psychopathy and physiological responses to threat of an aversive stimulus. *Psychophysiology, 15*(2), 165–172. https://doi.org/10.1111/j.1469-8986.1978.tb01356.x

Harron, M., (Director). (2000). *American psycho* [film]. Lions Gate Films.

Harvey, P., Stoner, J., Hochwarter, W., & Kacmar, C. (2007). Coping with abusive supervision: The neutralizing effects of ingratiation and positive affect on negative employee outcomes. *The Leadership Quarterly, 18*(3), 264–280. https://doi.org/10.1016/j.leaqua.2007.03.008

Heilman, M. E. (2001). Description and prescription: How gender stereotypes prevent women's ascent up the organizational ladder. *Journal of Social Issues, 57*(4), 657–674. https://doi.org/10.1111/0022-4537.00234

Hicks, B. M., & Drislane, L. E. (2018). Variants ("subtypes") of psychopathy. In C. J. Patrick (Ed.), *Handbook of psychopathy* (2nd ed., pp. 297–334). Guilford.

Hurst, C., Simon, L., Jung, Y., & Pirouz, D. (2019). Are "bad" employees happier under bad bosses? Differing effects of abusive supervision on low and high primary psychopathy employees. *Journal of Business Ethics, 158*(4), 1149–1164. https://doi.org/10.1007/s10551-017-3770-5

Ishikawa, S. S., Raine, A., Lencz, T., Bihrle, S., & Lacasse, L. (2001). Autonomic stress reactivity and executive functions in successful and unsuccessful criminal psychopaths from the community. *Journal of abnormal psychology, 110*(3), 423–432. https://doi.org/10.1037//0021-843x.110.3.423.

Kelly, J. (2019, December 4). *How to tell if you work for a sociopath or psychopath.* Forbes. https://www.forbes.com/sites/jackkelly/2019/12/04/how-to-tell-if-you-work-for-a-sociopath-or-psychopath/?sh=1640a3d32b0c

Kupers, T. A. (2005). Toxic masculinity as a barrier to mental health treatment in prison. *Journal of Clinical Psychology, 61*(6), 713–724. https://doi.org/10.1002/jclp.20105

Landay, K., Harms, P. D., & Credé, M. (2018). Shall we serve the dark lords? A meta-analytic review of psychopathy and leadership. *Journal of Applied Psychology, 104*(1), 183–196. https://doi.org/10.1037/apl0000357

Lasko, E. N., & Chester, D. S. (2020). What makes a "successful" psychopath? Longitudinal trajectories of offenders' antisocial behavior and impulse control as a function of psychopathy. *Personality disorders.* Advance online publication. https://doi.org/10.1037/per0000421

Lilienfeld, S. O., Watts, A. L., & Smith, S. F. (2015). Successful psychopathy: A scientific status report. *Current Directions in Psychological Science, 24*(4), 298–303. https://doi.org/10.1177/0963721415580297

Lilienfeld, S. O., Smith, S. F., Sauvigné, K. C., Patrick, C. J., Drislane, L. E., Latzman, R. D., & Krueger, R. F. (2016). Is boldness relevant to psychopathic personality? Meta-analytic relations with non-psychopathy checklist-based measures of psychopathy. *Psychological Assessment, 28*(10), 1172–1185. https://doi.org/10.1037/pas0000244

Lykken, D. T. (1995). *The antisocial personalities.* Lawrence Erlbaum Associates, Inc.

Mathieu, C., & Babiak, P. (2016). Validating the B-scan self: A self-report measure of psychopathy in the workplace: B-scan self. *International Journal of Selection and Assessment, 24*(3), 272–284. https://doi.org/10.1111/ijsa.12146

Mathieu, C., Hare, R. D., Jones, D. N., Babiak, P., & Neumann, C. S. (2013). Factor structure of the B-scan 360: A measure of corporate psychopathy. *Psychological Assessment, 25*(1), 288–293. http://dx.doi.org.ezproxylocal.library.nova.edu/10.1037/a0029262

Mathieu, C., Neumann, C. S., Hare, R. D., & Babiak, P. (2014). A dark side of leadership: Corporate psychopathy and its influence on employee well-being and job satisfaction. *Personality and Individual Differences, 59*, 83–88. https://doi.org/10.1016/j.paid.2013.11.010

Moss-Racusin, C. A., Phelan, J. E., & Rudman, L. A. (2010). When men break the gender rules: Status incongruity and backlash against modest men. *Psychology of Men & Masculinity, 11*(2), 140–151. https://doi.org/10.1037/a0018093

Mullins-Sweatt, S. N., Glover, N. G., Derefinko, K. J., Miller, J. D., & Widiger, T. A. (2010). The search for the successful psychopath. *Journal of Research in Personality, 44*(4), 554–558. https://doi.org/10.1016/j.jrp.2010.05.010

Omar, A. M. A., Wisniewski, T. P., & Yekini, L. S. (2019). Psychopathic traits of corporate leadership as predictors of future stock returns. *European Financial Management, 25*(5), 1196–1228. https://doi.org/10.1111/eufm.12244

Palmen, D. G. C., Derksen, J. J. L., & Kolthoff, E. (2020). High self-control may support 'success' in psychopathic leadership: Self-control versus impulsivity in psychopathic leadership. *Aggression and Violent Behavior, 50*, 101338. https://doi.org/10.1016/j.avb.2019.101338

Patrick, C. J., Fowles, D. C., & Krueger, R. F. (2009). Triarchic conceptualization of psychopathy: Developmental origins of disinhibition, boldness, and meanness. *Development and Psychopathology, 21*(3), 913–938. https://doi.org/10.1017/S0954579409000492

Pech, R. J., & Slade, B. W. (2007). Organisational sociopaths: Rarely challenged, often promoted. Why? *Society and Business Review, 2*(3), 254–269. https://doi.org/10.1108/17465680710825451

Perri, F. S. (2011). White-collar criminals: The 'kinder, gentler' offender?: White-collar crime, fraud, offender. *Journal of Investigative Psychology and Offender Profiling, 8*(3), 217–241. https://doi.org/10.1002/jip.140

Perri, F. S. (2013). Visionaries or false prophets. *Journal of Contemporary Criminal Justice, 29*(3), 331–350. https://doi.org/10.1177/1043986213496008

Perri, F. S., & Lichtenwald, T. G. (2010). The last frontier: Myths & the female psychopathic killer. *Forensic Examiner, 19*(2), 50.

Persson, B. N., & Lilienfeld, S. O. (2019). Social status as one key indicator of successful psychopathy: An initial empirical investigation. *Personality and Individual Differences, 141*, 209–217. https://doi.org/10.1016/j.paid.2019.01.020

Pheko, M. M. (2018). Rumors and gossip as tools of social undermining and social dominance in workplace bullying and mobbing practices: A closer look at perceived perpetrator motives. *Journal of Human Behavior in the Social Environment, 28*(4), 449–465. https://doi.org/10.1080/10911359.2017.1421111

Phelan, J. E., Moss-Racusin, C. A., & Rudman, L. A. (2008). Competent yet out in the cold: Shifting criteria for hiring reflect backlash toward agentic women. *Psychology of Women Quarterly, 32*(4), 406–413. https://doi.org/10.1111/j.1471-6402.2008.00454.x.

Player, A., Randsley de Moura, G., Leite, A. C., Abrams, D., & Tresh, F. (2019). Overlooked leadership potential: The preference for leadership potential in job candidates who are men vs. women. *Frontiers in Psychology, 10*, 755. https://doi.org/10.3389/fpsyg.2019.00755

Pletti, C., Lotto, L., Buodo, G., & Sarlo, M. (2017). It's immoral, but I'd do it! Psychopathy traits affect decision-making in sacrificial dilemmas and in everyday moral situations. *British Journal of Psychology, 108*(2), 351–368. https://doi.org/10.1111/bjop.12205

Poythress, N. G., & Hall, J. R. (2011). Psychopathy and impulsivity reconsidered. *Aggression and Violent Behavior, 16*(2), 120–134. https://doi.org/10.1016/j.avb.2011.02.003.

Ragatz, L. L., Fremouw, W., & Baker, E. (2012). The psychological profile of white-collar offenders: Demographics, criminal thinking, psychopathic traits, and psychopathology. *Criminal Justice and Behavior, 39*(7), 978–997. https://doi.org/10.1177/0093854812437846

Rilling, J. K., Glenn, A. L., Jairam, M. R., Pagnoni, G., Goldsmith, D. R., Elfenbein, H. A., & Lilienfeld, S. O. (2007). Neural correlates of social cooperation and non-cooperation as a function of psychopathy. *Biological Psychiatry, 61*(11), 1260–1271. https://doi.org/10.1016/j.biopsych.2006.07.021

Rose, K., Shuck, B., Twyford, D., & Bergman, M. (2015). Skunked: An integrative review exploring the consequences of the dysfunctional leader and implications for those employees who work for them. *Human Resource Development Review, 14*(1), 64–90. https://doi.org/10.1111/j.1464-0597.2006.00226.x

Sellbom, M., & Drislane, L. E. (2020). The classification of psychopathy. *Aggression and Violent Behavior, 101473*. https://doi.org/10.1016/j.avb.2020.101473

Skeem, J. L., Polaschek, D. L. L., Patrick, C. J., & Lilienfeld, S. O. (2011). Psychopathic personality: Bridging the gap between scientific evidence and public policy. *Psychological Science in the Public Interest, 12*(3), 95–162. https://doi.org/10.1177/1529100611426706

Smith, S. F., & Lilienfeld, S. O. (2013). Psychopathy in the workplace: The knowns and unknowns. *Aggression and Violent Behavior, 18*(2), 204–218. https://doi.org/10.1016/j.avb.2012.11.007

Spencer, R. J., & Byrne, M. K. (2016). Relationship between the extent of psychopathic features among corporate managers and subsequent employee job satisfaction. *Personality and Individual Differences, 101*, 440–445. https://doi.org/10.1016/j.paid.2016.06.044

ten Brinke, L., Kish, A., & Keltner, D. (2018). Hedge fund managers with psychopathic tendencies make for worse investors. *Personality and Social Psychology Bulletin, 44*(2), 214–223. https://doi.org/10.1177/0146167217733080

Verona, E., & Vitale, J. (2018). Psychopathy in women: Assessment, manifestations, and etiology. In C. J. Patrick (Ed.), *Handbook of psychopathy* (pp. 509–528). The Guilford Press.

Wall, T. D., Sellbom, M., & Goodwin, B. E. (2013). Examination of intelligence as a compensatory factor in non-criminal psychopathy in a non-incarcerated sample. *Journal of Psychopathology and Behavioral Assessment, 35*, 450–459. https://doi.org/10.1007/s10862-013-9358-1

Waller, R., Gardner, F., & Hyde, L. W. (2013). What are the associations between parenting, callous-unemotional traits, and antisocial behavior in youth? A systematic review of evidence. *Clinical Psychology Review, 33*(4), 593–608. https://doi.org/10.1016/j.cpr.2013.03.001

Whitbourne, S. K. (2015, September 12). 20 signs that your boss may be a psychopath. *Psychology Today*. https://www.psychologytoday.com/us/blog/fulfillment-any-age/201509/20-signs-your-boss-may-be-psychopath

Whiteside, S. P., & Lynam, D. R. (2001). The five factor model and impulsivity: Using a structural model of personality to understand impulsivity. *Personality and Individual Differences, 30*(4), 669–689. https://doi.org/10.1016/S0191-8869(00)00064-7

Widom, C. S. (1977). A methodology for studying noninstitutionalized psychopaths. *Journal of Consulting and Clinical Psychology, 45*(4), 674.

Index

© The Author(s), under exclusive license to Springer Nature Switzerland AG 2021
T. D. Kennedy et al., *Working with Psychopathy*, SpringerBriefs in Psychology,
https://doi.org/10.1007/978-3-030-84025-9